THE
7
STEPS
TO OVERCOMING ARTHRITIS

By
Gary Null

ibooks
new york
www.ibooks.net

DISTRIBUTED BY SIMON & SCHUSTER, INC.

ibooks, inc.
24 West 25th Street
New York, NY 10010

The ibooks World Wide Web Site Address is:
http://www.ibooks.net

ISBN 0-7434-5891-5
First ibooks, inc. printing June 2003
10 9 8 7 6 5 4 3 2 1

Cover design by Carrie Monaco

Printed in the U.S.A.

ALSO AVAILABLE FROM IBOOKS, INC.:

The 7 Steps to Perfect Health
by Gary Null

The 7 Steps to Overcoming Depression and Anxiety
by Gary Null

Contents

INTRODUCTION

THIS is a book about arthritis. My goal is to offer you a full, effective, and practical approach to dealing with this terrible and widespread affliction. While it is true that an estimated 40 million Americans have one of the two main forms of the disease, osteo- or rheumatoid arthritis, or one of 100 related disorders, such as fibromyalgia, lupus, gout, or scleroderma, this fact will seem unimportant to the person who first experiences arthritic pains—or indeed, pains which he or she cannot identify at all. And yet there are some things common to us all, which slowly but surely lead to a myriad of conditions, among them arthritis. Finding this common background is crucial to understanding fully why a person develops this disease and what must be done to prevent it or else to reverse its painful symptoms and banish it forever.

In my book, *The Seven Steps to Perfect Health*, I outlined seven steps to ridding your body of stress and toxins so that you can enjoy a life of well-being and boundless energy. Those seven steps can be applied to any disease or condition, such as anxiety, depression, cardiovascular disease, obesity, or arthritis, to name just a few.

Step #1. Beginning the Road to Wellness—The first step to overcoming arthritis is to trace the problem to its source. In searching for the roots of arthritis in Chapter 1, The Common

Roots of the Problem, I will begin with a scenario that may at first glance seem to take us far from the subject at hand but will soon show us that health, illness, and aging are processes created by the choices we make.

Step #2. Eliminating Disease-Causing Agents—What can be done to prevent the inflammatory processes that lead to disease? What will heal the body from years of neglect? In Chapter 2, I will explain in detail why moderation in all things is not the best policy.

Step #3. Cleansing and Detoxifying for Strength and Stamina—A logical, safe, and holistic approach to cleansing and detoxifying indicates three main tasks: Remove the accumulated toxins in the body, build up the immune system, and give the body what it needs for optimal maintenance as well as emergencies. That is a very wide overview. There are, naturally, many separate tasks within these three and I will detail them all.

Step #4. Eating Well is the Best Revenge—The recipes in Chapter 6 are specially designed for the arthritic condition, and are easy enough for you to begin to incorporate into your diet and lifestyle.

Step #5. Exercise for Rejuvenation—No matter how much of this book you follow, if you don't begin a regimented program of exercise, your results will be minimal. Chapter 5 covers a complete protocol for the arthritic condition. The most important elements of this protocol are: eliminating possible food allergens, exercise, and juicing.

Step #6. De-Stressing Your Life—In any illness, stress is a real problem and a thorough stress-reduction regimen is essential. There are many different methods to choose from.

Step #7. Taking Charge of Your Perfect Heath—Only through hard work can we change bad habits and reach our health potential. I consider allegorical statements from clients and study members to be valid evidence of the success of my programs. I hope that the testimonials I've gathered from arthritis suffers will serve as inspiration and that you will soon add a testimonial of your own!

1

THE COMMON ROOTS
OF THE PROBLEM

LET us assume that there is such a phenomenon as an average person and that you are one of them. You are on your lunch break, looking at a menu. You don't have a lot of time. You are working in a very fast-paced office and you are under a lot of pressure. You once thought that when you grew up, you would have security, as your parents or grandparents possibly had, but things did not work out that way. You have watched as many of your colleagues have been fired and positions downsized. Companies like yours have been bought up by larger companies and stripped bare of assets, including the workforce. So each day when you go to work you are glad that, at least for the moment, you are making enough money to maintain your standard of living, but there is always that doubt that you will not be able to continue maintaining it. What if you tried your best, but nevertheless lose value to the company? What if the company simply does not care what happens to you?

So here you are, rushing to eat lunch. You are not thinking about sitting and enjoying the meal. The décor in American fast-food restaurants consists of colors, music, and furniture that are not meant for comfort. They are almost intentionally annoying, with their bright yellows, oranges, reds, loud music, and commercials. All these things, together with the noisy crowds, are quite irritating. Far more important than the ambiance is the food you are going to consume! You are going to eat it because it tastes good and you are very used to it. It fills you up, and from your point of view it is relatively inexpensive. Then you go back to work.

During the workday you will make a few concessions to your own needs, like making a few personal calls or sharing complaints with colleagues. In general though, you will work hard while looking forward to going home and turning on the television. Generally these are behavior patterns to which you have become accustomed. If you are married or with an essential other, you will more often than not share much of what happened during the day, including your frustrations. There is some empathizing, and then of course there is food. The pace is generally a little slower than at work, but not by too much, especially if there are evening plans.

You do not really focus on the evening meal, which is of secondary importance. True, you are hungry, but you want to eat quickly so you can lie down on the couch and watch television or go out and do something. Later, when you go to bed, you are generally a little bit congested and more than a little bit "hyper."

As an average American (which we are making believe you are), you will wake up in the morning constipated, full of mucous, bloated, puffy, and not completely rested. Then the routine starts all over again: You gulp down some sort of breakfast and rush out the door so your commute will get you to work on time. These average daily cycles are relatively the same, whether you are a factory worker, office worker, union, non-union, or a white- or blue-collar worker. It does not seem to matter.

Then there are the so-called upwardly mobile people. They

don't eat at fast-food restaurants but generally at one of the "better watering holes." I recently spoke with people at a few of these places in New York, Los Angeles, Chicago, Boston, and Washington, D.C. My guide pointed out the type of person who frequented various locales. For example, at Washington restaurants of this type were the go-getter lawyers from government bureaucracies who were always looking for "deals."

In fact, with this group, everybody seems to be looking for deals. Their actual work almost seems of secondary importance to what it gets them, like connections that can open doors. These are mini-power lunches and dinners. Generally alcohol is present—not to get people drunk, but to loosen them up. Their conversation is generally loud, designed to let off steam and to vent. The food is considered more upscale gourmet food, dishes like prime beef, pheasant, or exotic chicken, but not hamburgers and hotdogs. Those are saved for the weekend and the backyard.

These lives seem to be especially intense. For example, once or twice a week people of this social class go to the health club, and it is not for messing around, but for hard workouts. Almost everything in their life is based upon security and getting ahead while they still can. They generally tend to be more conscious of style and social position. A lot of drugs and medications are taken in this particular culture. For all intents and purposes, these people are completely functional, frequently look very fit, and are generally well educated. So unless you get close enough to see the defects, they are not always apparent.

Senior citizens form another subgroup among average Americans. Perhaps you are a member of this group, either widowed, single, or married. According to your economic status and desires, you may have already migrated to a warmer climate for the wintertime, to southern California, southern Texas, Arizona, or

Florida. Whether you live in a gated community with tennis, golf, or boating, or in a less affluent neighborhood, you will generally stick to the same daily routine so closely that it can be called a ritual. And this ritual will, more frequently the older you become, involve medical intervention and medications. It may also, for the average American, demonstrate a slightly increased awareness of health issues. For example, a senior citizen today will quite possibly take a one-a-day multi-vitamin and cut coffee drinking from two cups down to one at breakfast, and they may take walks or play golf a couple of times a week.

Americans love ritualistic living. It is extremely hard for us to change these rituals, even when it is to our great benefit to do so. If you are used to waking up in the morning, watching television, having coffee and a bagel; sugar-coated cereal and a cup of coffee; or a glass of orange juice and sugary cereal, it will be close to impossible to change that or any other type of lunch, dinner, or snack you habitually have. One need only think of the widespread habit of buying popcorn before seeing a movie. Unless there is a long concession line or you are late and the picture has started, nothing can stop you from buying that popcorn.

Another group of Americans, an unfortunate group, are those who are homebound. They may not need a nursing home or assisted living, and this is certainly an advantage, but these people are very lonely. They live in a limited environment without much social contact. Television, radio, and books take up their day, and, while these can be extremely stimulating, the fact remains that emotionally these people are looking at the world as if they are no longer a part of it. It is as if they are angels looking down at those still living and musing over what everyone is doing.

What do these descriptions of the various types of lives led by some average groups of Americans have to do with arthritis? Let us first discover what they have to do with ill health, immune system breakdown, and aging in general. After that, the development of arthritic conditions will fall into place.

These scenarios show that your life is made up of many decisions. I would like to suggest that every one of these choices, no matter how small or inconsequential it may seem, has a consequence, and in time these results add up to a noticeable condition. It is as if you are given a health bank account at birth. Withdrawals and deposits are often made in increments so small they seem to make no difference to your overall health balance. Of course they do add up eventually, and a general tendency toward robust health or illness becomes apparent. For example, each time you do something harmful to your health, a withdrawal, even if only a microscopic one, occurs, bringing you that much closer to health insolvency. By contrast, each good thing for your health brings a slight increase in your health balance. Of course, reality is not that simple. Some decisions affect whole interrelated body systems and cause quantum leaps, either positive or negative, in your health status.

The fact is that health is a lifelong, ongoing process. Illness and aging, therefore are processes as well.

For example, let us take the case of some friends in their 30s sitting in a bar talking about their joys, expectations, passions, and frustrations. They are drinking, but only an amount that allows them to maintain their composure and not feel drunk. Their internal biochemistries are the last thing on their minds. They are simply feeling the effect of the alcohol. They feel warm, more open, and expressive. It is becoming easier to talk, easier to get rid of some inhibitions and speak honestly. Nonetheless, developments are taking place within each of their bodies. With every drink they are contributing to an inflammatory process in their brains, kidneys, livers, and hearts. Enjoyments such as these young people are experiencing are fine, except that sometimes they are not fine for their cells.

THE TELOMERE, YOUR MOLECULAR CLOCK

Since we are made up of cells, if we are interested in our own aging and lifespan, we have to realize that each of our cells also has a lifespan and aging process. For obvious reasons, our lifespan and aging process and those of our cells are intimately connected!

The cell's lifespan is measured in divisions (the cell divides and replicates itself). Each cell is normally given a certain number of divisions, about 60 on average, before it reaches "replicative senescence" and then death. This may not sound like very many divisions, but actually 60 to 80 healthy cell divisions, each taking about 2½ years, would mean that theoretically and biologically the human body could live for 120 to 150 years. We are not even living half that long! The average lifespan for men in the United States is still under 75 years, with the last 25 being years of sickness. To be blunt, from the age of 50 on, most men are in varying stages of death because body systems have declined substantially.

There are 46 chromosomes in each cell. At each end of every chromosome is a structure made of DNA called a telomere. (There are 92 telomeres in each cell.) It is a sort of cap to protect the end of the chromosome from damage. Telomere DNA has over 1,000 bases, or tiny building blocks, with the repeating gene sequence TTAGG. In order to divide 100 percent accurately, the cell has to replicate all the DNA in its chromosomes. Normal cells are somehow not able to copy the last few building blocks of the telomere. As a result, the telomere shortens with each DNA replication and cell division. In observing this, we are looking in on the exact moments and locations of aging, when the cell does not reproduce accurately!

There comes a time, different for each person, cell, and chromosome, when the telomere can no longer shorten. At that point, a message goes out that says: "This cell has reached the end of its life. Start the process of an orderly suicide." Thus, as your telomeres shorten and cells die, you will not have the same muscle mass as before, or the same vision, neuron activity, or libido.

The telomere has been called a molecular clock. In a sense, it determines the age of your cell, constantly sending signals which tell the cell how long it is going to live, based on how much of the telomere is left. This is not the place to go into the many complexities of cellular research, such as the definite possibility of elongating the telomeres to add longevity to the cell, or the innate intelligence that the cell seems to have which allows it to modify gene expression during its lifetime, if given a chance. Suffice it to say that each of your cells at birth has a death date. If you do things in your life which increase the speed at which cell division occurs, that cell's death date may occur earlier, since the telomeres will shorten earlier and the given number of cell divisions will be reached sooner.

Because of this and many other factors, no two cells age at the same rate, not even if they are in the same organ! Therefore, aging is not uniform within a person. That is why you find people whose heart and lungs are functioning, but whose brain has deteriorated, or vice versa. In general, the skin will age before the muscles, which in turn age before the kidneys.

To put it another way, the benchmark of aging is the precipitous loss of cell function—that is, a rapid increase in the number of dead or dying cells which can no longer perform their tasks. DNA damage from many different causes results in a shortening of the telomeres, and cells divide in a shorter time span than the normal 2½ year period.

To explain it a third way, let us assume your life is a motion picture of three hours duration at normal speed. Because of your actions you have increased the movie projector's velocity so that the entire movie will now take only 45 minutes. In a panic, you yell out: "Hold on a second! Slow down!" Your cell says: "I can't. You're not helping me." You scream in despair: "Well, I don't want to die faster!" The cell replies: "Sure you do! You're doing nothing to stop it! If you keep on with this DNA damage, you're going to go even faster. You've got to stop making excuses for what you are eating, and for your negative thoughts which make you angry, bitter, selfish, inconsiderate, apathetic, mean-spirited, and greedy. So you're going to be rewarded! After all, you've worked very hard at being sick!"

Many people, if they are honestly self-observant, should see themselves as having some of those base emotions listed above as well as bad dietary habits while functioning well on the surface. Yes, we are an extraordinarily functional society, but we live a very dysfunctional existence within that functional framework. It seems complicated only to us. To the cell it is simply a matter of getting the right tools so it can honor the body it is in. If it does not receive these tools, then the cell does the best it can with a bad bargain. The cell does not care if you eat dairy foods and meat every day of your life. It just records the DNA damage. The cell does not care what you are angry about, what you complain about, feel uptight or anxious about. "You didn't have sex last night and feel lousy about it? Okay. More DNA damage," says the cell, and you pay the price.

Young people drinking out of frustration at not getting success in life quickly enough are not helping their telomeres. Their chromosomes have been damaged. They are going to die faster. Senior citizens watching television scenes of activities which they used to do but never will again, and feeling despair about this are, sadly, dying faster as well.

Children often cannot articulate their pain, but their cells record it nevertheless. A "supermom" may be trying to balance raising a family with being the CEO of a company and getting everything out of life that she possibly can. She can afford to hire around-the-clock caretakers for her children. Quite possibly she will leave casualties along the way, such as dysfunctional children who hate her because of her lack of attention. The child may think: "My God! I never wanted to be born, especially not to you. You may be a supermom at achieving. You're not a super human being, a spiritual model for me to follow." The child doesn't know how to voice that. All the child can do is feel incompetent. However, the child's cells know just what to do. They start the death process.

Is that statement overly dramatic? Not really. The fact is, we are seeing diseases of old age in children now. And the parents who want acknowledgment for their "sacrifices" but do not get it suffer as well, and shorten their lives. When the average person eats a typical American breakfast consisting of orange juice, toast, eggs, sugary cereal, and coffee, does he actually ask himself: "Is this really what my body needs for maximal nutrition and vitality?" Probably not. Instead, most people say: "This is what I'm used to. This is what I like. I'm not going to change." And thus the assault on the cells continues.

Unfortunately, anything that is not supporting the health of the cell creates disease. The disease generally manifests first as an oxidative stress, which creates free radicals. The free radicals, which damage DNA and chromosomes, thus cause an alteration in what the cell does. The cell can no longer carry out its normal basic functions. And the damage in the cell then manifests as a glycation, an alteration in glucose.

The sugar in refined carbohydrates like pastas, fruit juices, white rice, white bread, bagels, cakes, candies, and cookies is so delicious that many people simply cannot live without it. The same addiction to dairy products is seen. This is most unfortunate, since sugar and dairy foods are major causes of sickness, including inflammatory arthritis. Little by little, almost imperceptibly, the disease processes take hold. Then "suddenly" one day you wake up with a noticeable symptom of a disease. And where inflammation has started, you will always find C-reactive protein.

C-REACTIVE PROTEIN

C-reactive protein is a molecule that is a primary indicator of inflammation, and inflammation is an immune response that occurs when something has been injured or where there is an infection, either bacterial or viral, or trauma. The outward signs are redness and swelling, which means that your immune system is working overtime to break down the injured and dying tissues so that new, healthy ones can replace them. This is a normal process. The production of C-reactive protein is an essential part of all inflammatory processes.

An astounding demonstration of the importance of C-reactive protein lies in the fact that if you do not check your C-reactive protein, you may have a 500 percent chance of dying of a heart attack, even if your cholesterol, triglycerides, and blood pressure are normal. You may think you are safe because you are not overweight, yet this does not seem to make a difference in this case.

You could still have an elevated C-reactive protein with a 500 percent chance of having cardiovascular disease and a 700 percent chance of having a heart attack or stroke.

Other causes of elevated C-reactive protein are the drug Premarin, high-protein diets, refined carbohydrates and sugars, carbonated beverages, artificial sweeteners, alcohol in any amount, being under stress, excess body fat, chronic periodontal conditions, arthritis in the knees, fibromyalgia, and asthma.

At this point, if you are used to the average American diet, you may very well think that there is simply nothing left for you to eat! However, we will show that not only is there a world of healthy, delicious food out there, but that you have the ability to select the foods, nutrients, beverages, and life processes that can reverse inflammatory process and bring down homocysteine, C-reactive protein, and fibrinogen levels. Unfortunately, we have found that indifference to our actions brings unpleasant rewards, namely, that in time your telomeres are going to get the message that you are not helping yourself and they will shorten prematurely, thus speeding up the death process.

Assuming that you are now no longer indifferent to your actions, we will show what to do to counter inflammatory process, and thus, arthritis, in the next chapters.

2

INFLAMMATORY PROCESSES:
THE FALLACY OF MODERATION

ARTHRITIS, fibromyalgia, heart disease, cancer, Alzheimer's disease, and dementia all have something in common: they are all disease *processes*. Every end-stage disease had to have a start, perhaps even years earlier. Before a house burns down, someone and something has to kindle the fire. The trouble is that in our lives we are not geared to thinking of processes, especially if they are subtle processes.

In fact, we are indifferent enough to believe that anything that is a subtle process is a non-process. We talk about moderation in all things. "As long as something is done in moderation, it cannot be that bad," we say. So our society actually encourages moderation in drinking, in eating meat, in displaying anger. This carries over into society's official view that pesticides and pollution in moderate amounts will not hurt.

Let us consider the logic behind that kind of thinking. It is well known that mercury in any amount is toxic, and that, like many things, it accumulates in the body over many years. Is it reasonable then to think of a moderate amount of mercury as somehow non-threatening or non-lethal to the system? There is a cause and effect for everything in life, and many little "deposits" and "withdrawals" really do add up in our "health bank account." "Don't sweat the small stuff" goes the saying. I would only add: "True, don't sweat it, for that would produce stress, but deal with the small stuff with knowledge and confident action in a manner that becomes routine and you don't even have to think too much about it. That way you will not wake up one day to a health emergency." Deal with the subtle processes of life.

On the following pages, I will deal with arthritis in a different way from that of the mainstream media or even so-called holistic nutritionists.

THE USUAL APPROACH

Forty to fifty million Americans are in pain. Sometimes the pain is so severe that it interferes a great deal with the quality of the sufferer's life. We have been led to believe that we cannot cure arthritic pain; we can only alleviate it at times by numbing the perception of the pain, or turning off some of the pain processes. The medications to do this are known as non-steroidal anti-inflammatories. One drug is called methyl prexate. At one time gold injections were popular. There are a host of other conventional treatments.

There is some lessening of the pain with these substances, but unfortunately there is no lessening of the disease process. In fact, it continues to get worse. If you have an arthritic joint in the knee or ankle and you put your foot up to rest it, this may help temporarily. But the minute you go back to walking, biking, or other activity, the pain will return.

CAUSES OF INFLAMMATION

Let us begin to name the things which may cause inflammation in our bodies. First, let us take a look at our environment. The pesticides on your produce, the artificial colorings and preservatives, the chlorine and fluoride in your tap water, the electromagnetic pulses that emanate from your television, computer, cell phone, hair dryer, microwave oven, electric blanket, and digital clock all create imbalances in your body. These are electrical, magnetic, hormonal, pH, and biochemical imbalances. It is not an exaggeration to say that our environment is a minefield! If we encounter the wrong thing—and it is almost impossible not to—an inflammatory process may start. The affected cells send signals, saying: "We are under attack!" A lot of potential damage is possible, since we have hundreds of trillions of cells!

PESTICIDES

Let us focus on one of these environmental hazards. Pesticides cannot be digested and metabolized properly. A pesticide, after all, is designed to end life, and that is exactly what it attempts to do in your body. It is there as a destructive agent, and, yes, it can get inside the cell. Once it pierces the cell's sensitive, fatty, semi-permeable membrane, it can attack the mitochondria, our energy factories. Luckily there are a lot of mitochondria in a given cell. But sooner or later, the chemical pesticide can adversely affect the mitochondria to the point that they can no longer produce enough energy to sustain that particular cell's life. Then it can go on to attack the chromosomes, which contain our genes.

It should be fairly apparent by now how essential it is to consume only organically-grown produce.

APOPTOSIS

Once the chromosomes and genes are damaged, the cell is really in a serious situation. Repair may not be possible. Some scientists believe that a cell knows when it is damaged and not properly repaired, and that if it continues to live, it will put out a defective message. If cell damage from free radicals, viruses, bacteria, microbes, and environmental pollutants reaches the chromosomes, and the damage is so bad that natural repair enzymes and proteins cannot fix it, then something very unusual and dramatic occurs: The cell commits suicide! The cell seems to sense that the damaged genes could end up causing cancer, which could be passed on to the next generation. So in an action reminiscent of the final scene of a tragic opera, in order to preserve the integrity of both the existing and future generations, the cell sacrifices itself. This process is called programmed cell death, or apoptosis. The principle event in this is the opening of the mitochondrial "megachannel" through which the remaining cell energy seeps out until the cell dies. It is a controlled and orderly, non-inflammatory process.

FIGHTING INFLAMMATIONS

Inflammations caused by free radicals from viruses, bacteria, and environmental toxins are extinguished, so to speak, by antioxidants, the body's firefighters. Of course, as in any combustible situation, they are not always able to put the flames out in time. While it is true that antioxidants trap different types of free radicals, an antioxidant will not be able to stop an actual chemical. The chemical causes more free radicals, and these free radicals in turn attack the cell. Since antioxidants cannot successfully fight a chemical invader per se, we need many extra antioxidants to fight the extra free radicals produced by chemicals. A strong overall immune system is crucial for this effort.

Included in our immune systems are little "Pac Man" type

organisms called phagocytes. They will go after and engulf pesticide particles and try to destroy them with enzymes. Afterward, glutathione and other nutrients remove them from the system. The remaining free radicals are mopped up by antioxidants like vitamin C, vitamin E, zinc, selenium, n-acetyl cysteine, grape seed extract, and glutathione, as well as green tea, bilberry extract, beta-carotene, and the sulfur amino acids lutein and cysteine.

Vitamin C is of course one of the supreme antioxidants. One reason for this is that it stimulates natural killer cell activity, which can help stop resistant viruses.

BUYING PRODUCE IS SERIOUS BUSINESS

It is tragic, but well-intentioned people will go through their lives killing themselves slowly by not understanding that anything—yes, anything—that is non-constructive to life is automatically destructive. As stated earlier, it is the small things which you should be concerned about because you only get a big problem when the small problems accumulate. The cells are indeed extremely small! But if they could talk they might tell you that small things, such as buying conventionally-grown produce, are large, important, life-and-death concerns. With this consideration I urge you to buy all-organic foods exclusively.

Realize that the average non-health food consumer is buying known cancer-causing agents (of which there are hundreds sprayed on foods) as well as foods deficient in nutrients because of the artificial fertilizers used to grow them. (This food also lacks vital force, but that is an esoteric, but important, measurement.) We must first realize that our consumer habits are based on beliefs, not facts. If we could turn this around, the food we choose would be very different.

MEAT

Pesticides are just one of many terrible substances which enter our systems. Sadly, we take many deleterious foods for granted, and reach for them automatically.

As John Travolta's character was saying to Samuel Jackson's character in the movie *Pulp Fiction*, "Why are you eating pork?" "Well, because I like it. It tastes good," is the reply. "It's a diseased animal," Travolta's character counters. " I don't care," says Jackson's character. "I like it."

This typical disregard of one's own best interests is the first area of our psyche that needs to be observed. Observation and awareness can begin a cascade of inner changes.

EXCITOTOXINS AND OTHER POISONS

Almost everything in our society is done with the subtlety of a sledgehammer across rice paper. We have lost our capacity for subtlety. Everything today must be obvious to make its point. Our food is no exception. It is made to jolt us, titillate us, and make us swoon with sensory delight. But many of these substances, such as sugar and coffee, are poisons. They are jolts to the nervous system and to the cells. They are known as excitotoxins.

Highly refined and processed carbohydrates such as bread, muffins, and pastries are also assaults on the system. We frequently send our kids off to school after a breakfast of these excitotoxins and other dangerous substances. Then we give them lunches consisting of more of them. Why are we amazed that we get reports back from their teachers about our children bouncing off the walls? Then we allow the psychiatrist to diagnosis them as being brain disordered when they are really just hyper. These are normal kids on an abnormal diet.

We then drink tap water, which today is a garbage dump of toxic industrial chemicals, a definite assault on our cells. Throughout the day almost every single thing we take in has an adverse effect. Today it is possible to consume, in one day, about 150 artificial chemicals that have no place in the human body. All of that has to be dealt with by the body's biochemistry. And many of us just assume that our body's biochemistry is in good enough shape to fight on our behalf.

But sadly, that is not true. DHEA, the body's master hormone, declines substantially as we age. As DHEA declines, all of the processes it influences decline. As we get older, we are more likely to experience all forms of sickness, including inflammatory diseases. And every time we have sugar or caffeine or get excited, angry, nervous, or anxious in some way, we secrete stress hormones like adrenaline. We raise our blood sugar levels. Our bodies put out cortisol, and that causes inflammation.

The foods that we eat, and the chemicals on them, cause inflammation. Those people on a high protein diet are taking in unhealthy proteins, regardless of whether they lose weight or not. We take in mucous producing foods like dairy products and sugar. Sugar is a substance that, without a doubt, depresses the immune system because it depresses antibody activity.

On top of all this, we assume that everything we take in is going to be properly processed. Of course it is not, and we end up with something called a leaky gut, where toxins and undigested food particles actually wind up in the bloodstream.

We do not use proper dosages of supplements. We are deficient in virtually all the major nutrients. Many 50-year-olds suffer from the end stage of something they paid no attention to throughout their lives. The result of this inattention is inflammation.

Taken in total, dairy foods, wheat, sugar, meat, caffeine, carbonated beverages, artificial sweeteners, pesticides, herbicides, fungicides, and the electromagnetic pulses around us represent a full-frontal assault on the immune system.

And misleading measurements make it seem as if the assault is harmless. What could be bad about anything entering the body at parts per billion? The problem is that we are not just taking in one single item that has one single part per billion. People eat what they like in whatever amounts they choose: usually very large amounts. People do not eat based upon what their bodies need or how much they actually benefit from what they take in. Even if meat were somehow good for us, there would only be the need for about three ounces a day. Obviously, meat-eaters eat far more than that. If you asked a waiter for a three-ounce steak, he would not know what to give you. They do not even have children's portions that small! Due to misguided notions, an 80-year-old person with severe arthritis and an 18-year-old 200-pound athlete will get the same serving of steak! Does that make any kind of sense? Of course not. It is absurd.

MORE ON THE ORTHODOX APPROACH

Perhaps you are thinking: "Okay. I've got this inflammation. I've got stiff joints. Now I've got to adapt my life to this." But the mindset of adaptation is itself destructive in the context of how we proceed: We start excluding things from our life that at one time gave us pleasure, especially if they could cause us pain or swelling. But most of us will do nothing to learn about the underlying cause of the pain, or take steps to eliminate it.

Perhaps your doctor will make the usual orthodox statement that there is no cause and effect between what you eat and arthritis: "It is genetic. And if you don't believe me, call the Arthritis Foundation." End of discussion. Most doctors will tell you that there is no connection between what you eat and arthritis.

Are these doctors talking out of personal experience? Have they tried holistic regimens? Have they heard firsthand from patients who were helped by changing their eating habits? Probably not. Well then, are these doctors psychic? They seem so sure about their opinions.

THE ILLNESS CASCADE

People who have helped themselves recover from arthritis will tell you that allergies are a primary contributing factor to arthritic pain. Once you are allergic to something, every time you consume that offending substance, whatever it may be, your immune system is thrown into a tailspin. The end result is inflammation.

Madison Avenue claims there are drugs which help with the immune system. In point of fact there are no drugs that actually enhance the total immune system and have no side effects.

Once your immune system is depressed there are many forces just waiting to proliferate in your body. Viruses like herpes, Epstein Barr, and cytomegalovirus, adenoid viruses, bacteria, and yeasts are propagated. These lead to chronic infections. With this undermining of your system, you get even sicker than you ordinarily would when confronted with a toxic situation, such as emotional or physical trauma.

The following are some stressful situations that produce a perfect medium for the proliferation of common viruses, bacteria, and yeast: emotional stress from overwork; relationship problems; fears of terrorism and other threats; heavy metals and other environmental toxins lodged in your body, such as lead, cadmium, mercury (as in your dental fillings); processed, denatured, and dead food.

If you get sick from any of the above situations, your illnesses could multiply and worsen in what can be called an illness cascade, complete with negative hormones. You will then get infections which lead to inflammations.

PREVENTION AND HEALING

The good news about an anti-arthritic program is that it helps the body as a whole because it turns off system-wide inflammation. This will help with the fight against cancer, Alzheimer's disease, and heart disease, among others.

EDTA chelation (kee-LAY-shon) therapy has long been known as a safe way to get rid of heavy metals in the body. It consists of 20 to 40 or more office visits to get intravenous drips of a man-made amino acid called ethylene diamine tetra-acetic acid, which binds with heavy metals and takes them safely out of the body. Known chiefly for its great benefits to the cardiovascular system, it is also wonderful for arthritis sufferers and, indeed, for helping regain good health in old age. Long considered controversial by the mainstream medical establishment, which is fearful of losing revenues that would otherwise go toward coronary bypass operations and the like, chelation therapy is perfectly safe if performed by board certified chelationists. These doctors must be careful to put zinc, manganese, and other important minerals back into the body because EDTA removes some needed minerals along with the toxic ones. A frightening, but false idea about chelation is that it causes osteoporosis by removing calcium (which it does.) While it removes calcium from places where it does not belong, such as soft tissues (arteries, joints and muscles) the lowering of the calcium level in the blood prompts the parathyroid gland to secrete parathormone, which helps put calcium back into the bones, making them harder than before. Another scare disseminated by chelation's foes is that it will ruin the kidneys. Here, too, if administered correctly, chelation actually improves kidney function.

In addition to chelation therapy, which is highly recommended, you should start an elimination program. This has two goals: 1. Eliminate all deleterious substances from the body, either all at once, or gradually. This could very well diminish any arthritic pains. But if not, go on to the second part: Take one substance at a time, and eliminate it for a period. Note any changes in your pain or other conditions. Then put it back and eliminate another substance. You must keep very accurate and honest records for this to work.

The first stage of the elimination program generally consists of eliminating anything which contributes to the body's load of toxins and things which we can fairly well expect to be allergenic. Many of the bad foods and substances will be outlined later in this book. They include all meat, dairy foods, coffee, refined sugar, fried foods, and highly processed foods in general. If you cannot eliminate them all at once, make a schedule of elimination that you think you can stick to. This is very important. Remember that the goal is to really prevent or eliminate arthritic conditions without dangerous drugs which, in any case, do not work well.

A special caution about consuming meat is necessary. Meat brings arachidonic acid into the body. This acid is a precursor to prostaglandin E2 (a bad prostaglandin) and the pro-inflammatory cytokine leukotriene B4. Thus, one can make a case for meat being a cause of arthritic inflammations. The same caution goes for ingesting highly refined carbohydrates (cakes and cookies), which are high on the glycemic index (the sugar content quickly enters the bloodstream.) These, too, can lead to arachidonic acid overload.

You should start taking anti-viral and anti-bacterial substances such as Echinacea, Pau d'arco, astragalus, St. John's wort, and quercetin. This frees the body up to start its healing process.

HEALING FOODS

I would like to encourage eating only foods that cleanse and detoxify.

Every single day you should make sure to have green chlorophyll juices, starting with one juice per day for the first week, two juices per day the second week, three for the third, and so on until you are drinking six glasses of juice a day at the end of six weeks. IMPORTANT! You must make sure that you are not taking any medications that would interfere with the green juices. Be sure to consult with your physician because Comadine and green juices do not go well together.

Make sure that you have at least one daily phytochemically packed juice of berries, such as cherries, cranberries, raspberries, strawberries, blueberries, and blackberries. Berries are a terrific aid against arthritis! In the morning, have a drink made of lemon, lime, grapefruit, aloe vera, and raw honey.

A great juice for alleviating arthritis is a combination of ginger-root, apple, zucchini, broccoli, cucumber, kale, and the cabbage family. In fact cabbage juice is one of the single best juices. For example, try a combination of 4 ounces of aloe vera, 10 ounces of cabbage juice, and 6 ounces of water. Another beneficial combination is the terrific star fruit with pineapple and grapefruit. It is rich in enzymes, chlorophyll, oxidants, and nutrients. Potato juice—yes, RAW potatoes are used!—has historically been a known aid against arthritis. Boneset is important for arthritis as well.

It is crucially important to eat fresh greens such as parsley, broccoli, brussels sprouts, kale, dandelion, watercress, and arugula, as well as romaine, green leaf and red leaf lettuces. All of these wonderful foods flood the body with chlorophyll, oxygen, superoxide dismutase, and phytoestrogens, which help to rebalance hormones that protect the body against inflammatory processes, and also chelate out heavy metals. It is a slow process but a safe process. The cells really respond to the chlorophyll's living energy. To add a meat-like flavor, you can pour a small amount of sunflower oil on the greens.

You must incorporate high quality fiber—about 50 grams a day—into the diet. It absolutely must be in a whole, unprocessed form: blueberries, cherries, strawberries, beans, oats, groats, millet, buckwheat, rye, brown rice, amaranth, quinoa, or spelt. (Cooking the grains is the only form of processing allowed. But sprouting grains is a very healthy alternative to cooking.) As we digest whole grains, beans, seeds, and nuts—not roasted, salted nuts but whole nuts like walnuts, almonds, pine nuts, and pistachios—we are flooding the body with healthy fiber. This will lower cholesterol, lower triglycerides, lower excessive imbalances in estrogen, and give us anti-inflammatory fatty acids.

It is suggested that you orally supplement your diet with omega-3 fish oils, borage seed oil, flaxseed oil, oil of primrose, and black currant seed oil. Taking these oils—approximately 1,500 to 2,000 milligrams a day—does your body an enormous service because these are the oils that help give us more prostaglandin E1, which is an important part of our body's immune system that turns off naturally inflammatory processes and blocks prostaglandin E2 from turning them on. In effect, these oils fight inflammation all over the body. In addition, a teaspoon of emulsified cod liver oil on an empty stomach in the morning is always good for you.

Another crucial move against arthritis is to rebalance the body's pH. Our bodies are predominantly alkaline, as opposed to acidic. Eliminating all refined sugars and acidic foods is a first step. Rebalancing the pH from acid to alkaline can help with gouty arthritis and joint pain.

Since our bodies are about 70 percent water, it is absolutely essential to drink only clean water. This is especially important for people with arthritic conditions, as I will explain in a moment. You should drink at least one gallon of liquid (water and juice) daily. The water must be pure, either distilled or spring water. The fresh juices count toward the total liquid daily intake of a gallon. It is always important to hydrate the body tissues, but with arthritis it is even more important because hydrating the tissues also increases the lubrication within the tissue. The water aids the body's ability to flush out debris in the lymphatic system (which has no pump) as well as in the regular circulatory system.

Healthy fats are the only ones we should be allowing in our bodies. When you eat a heavy meal your blood looks a lot like a milkshake. That appearance is due to an excess amount of bad fats. Foods with healthy fats include cold-pressed, extra virgin, organic olive oil, avocados, nuts and seeds. These fats benefit the entire body, not just the arthritic areas.

Electromagnetic pulses in our immediate environment should be eliminated or minimized. Use a cell guard on your cell phone or cordless phone. Keep your body a proper distance from all electrical appliances. Wherever possible keep at least 18 inches from the smaller appliances, and at least six feet away from a large one, such as a television. Do not ever use a microwave oven or an electric blanket.

ASPIRIN

As is well known today, fresh juices do many good things: turn off inflammation, chelate out toxins, thin the blood naturally, help lower cholesterol, flood the body with vital life forces and healing enzymes, and help stop bleeding. This last benefit may come in handy because of America's drug of choice: aspirin.

Unfortunately, it is a good bet that someone with arthritic pain is, at some point, going to take an aspirin. Aspirin is one of the most single dangerous substances you can use. Here is why: It can cause dizziness. It can cause ringing in the ears and intestinal bleeding. It destroys the body's antioxidants, especially vitamin C. It causes kidney damage and lowers immunity. When aspirin fails to work, people start using non-steroidal anti-inflammatories. There have been reports of deaths from these drugs. In addition, aspirin users end up with bleeding ulcers, peptic ulcers, and conditions of nausea, nervousness, and vomiting. Then, if the non-steroidal anti-inflammatories fail to work, they go on to use the synthetic hormone cortisone, taken internally as Prednisone. This has many side effects and can be deadly.

But we do not have to use aspirin. There are natural substances which do similar things, without any side effects whatsoever, except one: good health!

For example, sulfur stops inflammation. It is, therefore, advisable to eat plenty of sulfer-rich foods like raw garlic, onions, and shallots. Omega fatty acids lubricate the joints. We therefore recommend coldwater fish like trout, sardines, mackerel and tuna.

Other anti-arthritis foods include avocadoes, walnuts, and almonds, as well as sunflower, pumpkin, sesame, and chia seeds, sea vegetables like Kombu, wakami, nori, and sea palm, soy protein from tofu, miso, tempeh and soy milk because it is rich in methionine. It is desirable to have at least three servings of cruciferous vegetables a day. Apricots, butternut squash, and Brazil nuts are also to be included in the diet.

Rebalance the healthy bacteria in the intestine by taking a nondairy acidophilus. In addition, certain nutrients are known to help heal the joints and repair damage to the cartilage and the tissue. For example, take glucosamine sulfate at 500 milligrams twice a day, chondroitin sulfate at 500 milligrams twice a day, and vitamin C at 5,000 to 10,000 milligrams a day in divided doses and on a gradual basis. Start with 500 milligrams a day. Then go to 700 milligrams a day, then 1,000 milligrams and so on. Always divide the doses, so that if you were taking 1,000 milligrams of vitamin C, you might take 200 milligrams five times during the day. Make sure you use a good quality vitamin C, and make extra sure it is buffered, because if it is not, you will suffer from acid in digestion and gastric distress. Vitamin C is crucial to the healing process as well as stopping inflammation.

You should also take 500 milligrams of grape seed extract. It strengthens the collagen and supports capillaries and veins. Take approximately 1,000 to 1,500 milligrams of whole pressed flaxseed oil a day, about 1,000 milligrams of oil of primrose, three milligrams of boron to help reverse many of the symptoms of osteoarthritis, ten milligrams of silica, two milligrams of copper, manganese at five to ten milligrams, and potassium at about 200 to 300 milligrams. Juices contain a lot of potassium, as do olives.

Ideally, we should stick with a living foods diet, consisting of very little cooked food. It is hard, if not impossible to think of someone developing arthritis on such a regimen! Of course, grains should be cooked (although, as mentioned previously, they can be sprouted for ultra-healthy snacks.) Beans are, of course, cooked (after soaking them overnight) and fish are steamed or broiled lightly. Vegetables may be steamed. However, nothing should ever be cooked to excess, and, of course, there should never, ever be any deep-frying because it alters protein in a dangerous way and makes it very difficult to digest.

A good example of a live food which is also fun to eat is the date. This is one of the most healing of all fruits. We do not eat enough of them. Figs, another underused fruit, together with fig juice and fig paste, are natural healing agents. These are the kind of sweets we should be indulging in! Although it is not ideal food-combining, a living food "cookie" which tastes very similar to a junk-food cookie can be made simply by eating a dried fruit together with a nut or seed. For example, eat raisins with walnuts, or dates with almonds.

This combination, while not the best, will do no harm because both substances are raw and almost completely unprocessed. However, when highly processed sugar and protein react, it is one of the worst possible things for your heart, your brain, and your joints. Such a reaction is called glycation, and it can cause calcium to go into the soft tissue instead of bones, where it belongs. Vitamin K can help avoid glycation, but many people with arthritis have a vitamin K deficiency. It is very easy to get and we don't need more than about ten milligrams. We can get it in a simple supplement which also includes 400 to 800 units of vitamin D3. This is tremendous help for our joints and bones.

Take the superstar antioxidant vitamin E with gamma tocopherols and tocotrienols—generally 400 to 600 IUs daily. Vitamin E is very beneficial because it also enhances oxygenation. It is a methylating agent. Methylation helps prevent arthritis, inflammatory processes and destruction of tissue. It is no surprise that the multi-talented superstar coenzyme Q10 is needed here as well—generally at 300 milligrams or up.

Alpha lipoic acid (400 to 1000 milligrams) works inside and outside the cell, protecting the joints. Alpha lipoic acid fights free radicals, but even more importantly, it stimulates the production of glutathione, the single most important antioxidant in the body. Glutathione is very hard to absorb orally unless you take a reduced form, and even then it will not be absorbed in high amounts. But we badly need this super antioxidant, which seems to do more than almost any other substance, and is naturally created by the body. The body creates three primary antioxidants: glutathione, melatonin, and superoxide dismutase. We need to take nutrients which will stimulate the production of these primary antioxidants.

Glutathione is what the body actually uses to protect against free radicals, but it also acts like a sanitation worker who sweeps the debris and the dead cells out of the body.

Converting protein into energy places an extraordinary burden on the body's metabolism. It is an extremely toxic process, with byproducts like ammonia, nitrogen, and urea. These all have to be eliminated quickly, and we can be thankful that glutathione is there to do the job. It is truly the great sanitation worker. However, when the sanitation workers go on strike, the body becomes almost uninhabitable.

In summary, it is crucial to take nutrients which create glutathione, such as n-acetyl cysteine at 500 to 1,000 milligrams, alpha lipoic acid, and grape seed extract at 200 to 500 milligrams.

Other helpful substances are superoxide dismutase, one of the primary antioxidants, greatly needed by the system, and vitamin B3 (niacin), extremely important for arthritis. Niacinamide (almost as effective as niacin, for those who cannot tolerate niacin) should be taken before a meal, generally two to three times a day (150-300 milligrams.) Pantothenic acid (generally 500 milligrams) helps rebuild the adrenal system, and almost everybody with gout and arthritis has a burnt-out adrenal system from stress and worry. The rest of the B complex should be taken as follows: B6—about 100 milligrams, B2—25 to 500 milligrams, and B1—25 to 50 milligrams. Folic acid at 400 to 800 micrograms (mcg) is very important be cause it helps lower the body's homocysteine level and fights against inflammatory processes. In addition, take the bioflavonoid quercetin, generally at 1,000 milligrams a day.

Sea cucumber is very good at lubricating parts of the body. MSM (methyl sulfonyl methane)—about 1,000 milligrams, twice a day, gets more sulfur into the body. Bromelaine, a great enzyme, helps in the production of prostaglandin and helps reduce inflammation. (Take as directed on the bottle.) Calcium and magnesium, from citrate, generally at 1,500 milligrams, is good because it helps prevent bone loss. DMG (dimethyl glycine) helps stop damage in the joints. Take about 100 to 125 milligrams, perhaps three times a day. TMG (trimethyl glycine) chemically related to DMG, should be taken at 200 milligrams. Take selenium at about 200 micrograms a day. Also consider MGM3, which is made from mushrooms, at about 1,500 milligrams. Glutamine helps to rebuild the intestinal lining and allows for better absorption and utilization of all the nutrients. It is generally taken at about 3,000 or 4,000 milligrams.

Lycopene, found not only in tomatoes, but in other red fruit, is very important for the immune system. It helps the body in general, as well as lowering the cholesterol level. L-carnitine, at about

500 milligrams, helps the energy in the cells through the mito-chondria. People with arthritis generally have lowered cellular energy, especially in the inflamed areas.

I would also include Boswellia, an Ayurvedic herb, which is important in helping stop inflammatory processes, and the impor-tant Peruvian herb cat's claw, a superstar in the herb family. How-ever, pregnant women should not take cat's claw. Cayenne pepper, and, in fact, all of the hot peppers, have capsicum, which is an important substance for blocking pain in a natural way. You should experiment—carefully!—to see how much, and in what form, your body can best use these very useful herbs. Olive leaf extract is also good for arthritis, as is turmeric (an ingredient in curry powder) which has curcumin, which, among many good things, turns off inflammation and helps to rejuvenate the immune system. Nettle leaf, used as a tea or as a tincture, is an anti-inflammatory, as is willow bark. Boswellia is one of the most important herbs, used throughout the Middle East. It is a natural pain reliever, with no harmful side effects. Here are some other herbs to include: Bur-dock root, comfrey, prickly ash bark, yucca, horsetail, at about 25 milligrams, black cumin, as directed, camu-camu, and English walnuts.

DHEA is the most crucial single hormone in the body. I find that it is deficient in a lot of people with arthritis. It helps not just with arthritis, but with immune function, muscle wasting, low energy, and osteoporosis. A dose of between 25 to 50 milligrams will generally help most people.

We cannot overlook the care of the liver. The liver is a crucial organ. It is central to metabolism, detoxification, filtration, immune function and bowel production. The more toxic the liver is, the more toxic the entire body will be. When the liver malfunctions, the whole body is susceptible to a myriad of conditions.

Juicing helps the liver. The herb milk thistle is known to greatly help this organ. By putting lots of good quality vegetables and juices into the system you will help stimulate the liver.

OTHER THERAPIES AND EXERCISE

Homeopathic remedies for arthritis include Rhus toxicodendron, calcarea carbonica and aconitum hapellus.

Reconstructive therapy consists of injecting a saline solution into the ligaments, tendons and cartilage to help stimulate them. It can make a difference, but it is not a cure-all. Neuromuscular therapy has been beneficial, as has therapeutic touch and chiropractic care. Clean up the environment. Detoxify the body. Rejuvenate the cells.

It is generally very important to start exercising, even if it causes some pain. Exercising increases the detoxification of the body, which is one of our main goals. It enhances the endorphins in the brain and helps to move healing nutrients into the damaged areas, while also helping remove debris. It also oxygenates and rejuvenates the blood. The arthritis sufferer may be able to handle light exercises such as water aerobics, where pressure is taken off the joints and tendons. Power walking and biking should also be considered, if they do not cause too much pain. Try to exercise on a regular basis and build up to one hour daily.

3

WHAT'S WRONG WITH THE TRADITIONAL ALLOPATHIC APPROACH?

WHAT does the average patient do when diagnosed with a condition like rheumatoid arthritis? Their doctor may give them the latest anti-inflammation medication and a pamphlet from the Arthritis Foundation, which is funded by private donations, the government, and drug companies. They may even visit their website where the Arthritis Foundation's "Guide to Good Living with Rheumatoid Arthritis" and "Alternative Therapies" can be purchased. The site enthusiastically ensures them that these booklets will provide "updates on the latest drugs, surgical techniques and therapies; insight into how rheumatoid arthritis develops and affects the body; guidelines for managing weight, fitness and stress; and, much more!" The Arthritis Foundation homepage of the site features special links on "Joint Surgery Jitters" to answer their questions, where they can view surgery animations to calm their fears. It also recommends the new Joint Surgery Book. Their booklet "Drugs for Arthritis" lists non-steroidal anti-inflammatories (NSAIDs), Analgesics, Biologic Response Modifiers, Glucocorticoids, DMARDs (Disease Modifying Anti-Rheumatic Drugs),

Fibromyalgia Medications, Osteoporosis Medications, Gout Medications, plus a section called Rub It On: Topical Analgesics. It has chapters titled "Kids Need Medications, Too" and "Medical Alternatives: When Drugs Aren't Enough," and offers a Drug and Dosage Diary. It highlights new drug breakthroughs and offers a new arthritis drug free to seniors until the government picks up the tab.

Let's look at what you're getting when you take drugs for arthritis. The first drugs offered are simple analgesics or pain relievers, next come nonsteroidal anti-inflammatory drugs (NSAIDs), then corticosteroids, followed by cortisone injections. By far the most common drugs used by arthritic patients, or the public in general, are pain killers. Thirty billion dollars worth of pain relieving medication is sold each year for the 100 million people suffering from chronic pain. About 40 million of those individuals suffer from arthritis. Aspirin, ibuprofen (a non-steroidal anti-inflammatory NSAID), and acetaminophen (Tylenol) are sold over the counter and are the first medications that are used for the pain of arthritis. Because they are so freely available, most people think they are harmless. Nothing could be farther from the truth.

ASPIRIN

On the Aspirin Foundation website we learn that aspirin was the first, and is today the most widely used pain reliever in the world. Like many medications it originated as an herbal medicine whose properties were later synthesized in a lab. It is now the active ingredient in more than 50 over-the-counter medications. It's over 100 years old but it was only in 1971 that the mechanism of its action was found; it inhibits prostaglandins, which are chemicals that cause pain and inflammation. That discovery, by Sir John Vane, a British pharmacologist, won him a Nobel Prize.

Aspirin is used to treat various forms of pain caused by muscle strains, headaches, and arthritis. Aspirin also thins the blood and prevents blood clots and is approved by the FDA to prevent heart disease in people who have suffered a heart attack, a stroke, or who have angina. The plant that aspirin derives from is willow bark, which has been used for centuries, ground up and used in teas and tinctures for easing aches and pains. In 1897 a German chemist Felix Hoffman discovered salicin in willow bark and found that to be the most active ingredient. The first salicylates, as they were called, were very hard on the stomach and Hoffman, who was trying to find an arthritis medication for his father, synthesized acetylsalicylic acid (ASA) instead of extracting the medicine from willow bark.

The Aspirin Foundation of America was founded in 1981 to "serve as a central source of information on the health benefits of aspirin and aspirin products." But in the same paragraph the foundation says it does not "promote aspirin or aspirin-related products!" However, the Aspirin Foundation ushers in each new study touting the benefits of aspirin with considerable fanfare using press releases to the media. It also fires off press releases if its favorite product is being maligned. One especially interesting missive in January 1998 argued that the FDA's proposed alcohol warning on aspirin would "mislead consumers." The Aspirin Foundation says that there are not enough studies to show that aspirin along with alcohol causes more gastrointestinal (GI) bleeding. They also claim that the initiative for the labeling arose from their competition, the makers of Tylenol. There are many press releases attesting to the pitched battle with their competitors for market share. The foundation also makes sure people don't misinterpret studies that suggest aspirin is dangerous; one that links aspirin to chronic renal failure, they say, may be biased. And they promote studies that say "Aspirin is Underused."

In spite of the fact that the Aspirin Foundation is a source of information about aspirin, not once do they talk about its side effects. Dozens of contraindications, precautions, adverse effects, and interactions can be found in the *Physician's Desk Reference* (PDR). For example, aspirin use is contraindicated and precaution advised in the following conditions: acid/base imbalance, acute bronchospasm, agranulocytosis, alcoholism, anemia, anticoagulant therapy, ascites, asthma, bone marrow suppression, breast-feeding, coagulopathy, dehydration, elderly, esophagitis, G6PD deficiency, gastritis, GI bleeding, GI disease, gout, hemophilia, hepatic disease, hypertension, hypoprothrombinemia, hypovolemia, immunosuppression, influenza, intramuscular injections, iron-deficiency anemia, labor, metabolic acidosis, metabolic alkalosis, nasal polyps, neutropenia, peptic ulcer disease, pregnancy, renal disease, renal failure, renal impairment, respiratory acidosis, respiratory alkalosis, salicylate hypersensitivity, surgery, systemic lupus erythematosus (SLE), tartrazine dye hypersensitivity, thrombocytopenia, thrombolytic therapy, thrombolitic thromobocytopenic purpura (TTP), tobacco smoking, urticaria, varicella, viral infection, and vitamin K deficiency.

Aspirin's adverse reactions constitute another long listing in the *PDR*: abdominal pain, agranulocytosis, anaphylaxis, angioedema, aplastic anemia, azotemia, bleeding bronchospasm, confusion, constipation, dehydration, diaphoresis, diarrhea, disseminated intravascular coagulation (DIC), dizziness, drowsiness, dyspepsia, dysphagia, elevated hepatic enzymes, encephalopathy, erythema nodosum, esophageal stricture, esophageal ulceration, esophagitis, fever, gastritis, GI bleeding, hallucinations, headache, hearing loss, hemolytic anemia, hepatic necrosis, hepatitis, hyperbilirubinemia, hyperglycemia, hypernatremia, hyperuricemia, hyperventilation, hypoglycemia, hypokalemia, hypoprothrombinemia, interstitial nephritis, jaundice, leukocytosis, leukopenia, maculopapular rash, metabolic acidosis, nausea/vomiting, odynophagia, pancytopenia, peptic ulcer, platelet dysfunction, prolonged bleeding time, pulmonary edema, purpura, renal failure, renal papillary necrosis, renal tubular necrosis, respiratory depression, Reye's syndrome, rhinitis, seizures, Stevens-Johnson syndrome, thrombocytopenia, tinnitis, toxic epidermal necrolysis, urticaria, visual impairment, and wheezing.

Perhaps what we learn from this long and impressive list of adverse reactions is that because aspirin has been used by millions of people for over 100 years, we've had ample time for all its side effects to surface. Similarly, there is a long list of negative interactions with other drugs provided by the *PDR*. However, because so many people feel aspirin is harmless, no studies have been done to warn people. They find out the hard way that there are negative effects when taking aspirin with the hundreds of drugs in the following drug groups: Aminoglycosides, Angiotensin-converting enzyme inhibitors (ACE inhibitors), Antacids, Anticoagulants, Antidiabetic agents, Antineoplastic agents, Beta-blockers, Corticosteroids, Cyclosporine, Diuretics, Nonsteroidal anti-inflammatory drugs (NSAIDs), Penicillins, Photosensitizing agents, Platelet inhibitors, Salicylates, Sulfonamides, and Thrombolytic agents. Or when taking the following specific drugs, herbs, and vitamins with aspirin: Acetaminophen, Acetazolamide, Alendronate, Ammonium chloride, Amphotericin B, Antithymocyte globulin, Ascorbid acid, Bacitracin, Bismuth Subsalicylate, Cefamandole, Cefoperazone, Cefotetan, Cidofovir, Cisplatin, Ethanol, Feverfew, Fish oil, Omega-3 Fatty Acids, Flaxseed, Foscarnet, Fosphenytoin, Garlic, Ginger, Ginkgo, Horse chestnut, Methazolamide, Methotrexate, Mycophenolate,

Phenytoin, Prasterone-Dehydroepiandrosterone-DHEA, Probene-cid, Strontium-89 chloride, Sulfinpyrazone, Valproic acid, Vancomycin, and Varicella virus live vaccine.

For an industry to say that aspirin is their safest product for arthritis is chilling, especially when we know that there are alternatives that work and have few if any side effects.

Meanwhile, the aspirin industry continues to abuse medical consumers with even more potent products. The newest is called "super-aspirin." Even though it is not going to be used on those afflicted with arthritis, it is instructive to study the cynical testing and marketing of this particular drug in light of all the other drugs reviewed in this chapter. When testing began five years ago, researchers were optimistic that the drug would improve on the common 2-cent variety of aspirin, which is still the most important medicine for heart disease. But each study ended badly. So badly that some are demanding the pharmaceutical industry stop the testing because super-aspirin may actually kill more volunteers than it saves. Super-aspirin is in a class of blood thinner known technically as IIb/IIIa antagonist. It is already injected to keep blood vessels flowing smoothly after angioplasties and mild heart attacks. But the drug companies wanted to tap a larger market for this medicine in a new pill form. It is not to be confused with the cox-2 inhibitors, including Celebrex, used to treat arthritis and are also called super-aspirin sometimes. This super-aspirin is being designed to be taken by millions of people with bad hearts to ward off heart attacks, strokes and death. It was assumed it would be just like aspirin, only more effective—but, of course, a lot more expensive.

The companies have spent hundreds of millions to prove super-aspirin works as well in practice as it ought to in theory. About 42,500 volunteers have tested four slightly different kinds in five large studies and each time the outcome was the same. But Dr. Eric Topol, cardiology chief at the Cleveland Clinic and director of two of the studies, claims between 150 and 200 volunteers probably died from the treatment itself. Nevertheless, the testing continues, as DuPont Pharmaceutical enrolled 2,200 patients in North America and Europe to test their super-aspirin, roxifiban. However, a debate has broken out as cardiologists argue whether DuPont should let the study go on. Some consider the drug too dangerous to keep testing on people while others claim the study's risks will be slight if it is stopped at the first hint of trouble. The latter hold up the prospect the drug could be a life saver and it would be tragic to give up on the treatment since ordinary aspirin only reduces the risk of death from heart disease by about 20 percent.

Doubts that super-aspirin will ever live up to the hype have grown in the last couple of years. A committee of doctors met in Boston to review the data from BRAVO (Blockade of the IIb/IIIa Receptor to Avoid Vascular Occlusion), a big study of a super-aspirin called lotrafiban. This committee's role was to make sure the study was not hurting anyone and it worked independently of the study's lead doctors and corporate sponsor, SmithKline Beecham. It was permitted to look at the ongoing results, which the other doctors involved could not do. This study involved 9,200 patients on four continents. Such large numbers are necessary to reveal small effects of the drug. The numbers showed that the death rate was actually higher among the volunteers getting lotrafiban—2.7 percent compared to 2 percent in the people taking "dummy pills." This amounted to 30 extra deaths among the lotrifiban users—30 deaths that may have been caused by the drug itself. Committee members wondered if the drug was truly to blame because two weeks earlier the number of deaths in the two groups was the same. One committee member, Dr. James Tcheng of Duke University, said, "If this had been the first time through with an oral IIb/IIIa antagonist, we might not have stopped the trial. We would have assumed that it might have been just a blip." But this was not the first time through. It was the fifth. And each study showed essentially the same thing: more deaths in people taking super-aspirin.

It was time to stop BRAVO. The committee sent a letter to the 700 hospitals in 30 countries with patients in the study urging them to take the patients off the drugs. Topol, the study's chairman, signed the letter. This was the second bad experience for him since he had earlier headed a study called SYMPHONY, looking at Roche's sibrafiban, which also ended in failure. Topol combined the five big studies and found that taking super-aspirin increased people's risk of death by 36 percent. It seemed that many of the extra deaths were cardiac arrests, which may have been triggered by blood clots, the very thing super-aspirin is supposed to prevent. IIb/IIIa antagonists are widely used and considered highly effective, in their injected form, as they subdue platelets, the blood cells that form clots. When injected, the drugs can stifle platelets' tendency to clump together by 90 percent or more. Since the risk of dangerous clots is especially high in some hospital situations, this is very useful. But the probability of unintended and possibly disastrous bleeding is too high to continue this treatment indefinitely. The pill form is less powerful, inhibiting platelets about 50 percent. Still, it is potent medicine, and it seemed logical it would help people with serious heart disease, misguided clots being the primary trigger of strokes and heart attacks. "Everybody thought this would be the next zillion-dollar drug," said Dr. John Ambrose of St. Vincent's Hospital in New York City.

* * *

Even though nobody knows why these disastrous results are occurring, several theories are being proposed. One is that super-aspirin triggers heart cells to commit suicide. Another speculates that it sets off a wave of inflammation. The leading theory says that the pills fail because of their halfway action and it appears that disabling the body's clot-making machinery this way is a bad idea. The drug works by sticking to the fibrinogen receptor, blocking the spot on the surface of platelets that ordinarily lets in chemical signals telling them to form clots. After someone takes a pill, the amount of medicine in the bloodstream gradually falls until it's time to take another one. As these drug levels grow low, more and more of the platelets' fibrinogen receptors are uncovered. But the cells do not like to have their receptors blocked and then reopened this way. It leaves them in a hair-trigger state, ready to clump into clots with little provocation. So as a result, many researchers think super-aspirin has a paradoxical effect: simultaneously inhibiting and activating platelets. The net effect is more clots, not fewer.

Still, Topol cautions that no one knows for certain why the first four super-aspirins tested were dangerous. Therefore, "I think there should be a moratorium on this drug class," he says. "At this point, I think it's unethical to continue the PURPOSE trial." PURPOSE is DuPont Pharmaceutical's study of roxifiban, the only super-aspirin pills now in human testing. Eventually the PURPOSE doctors voted to keep going, but with one major change: they would tighten the guidelines for stopping the study at the first hint of unexpected deaths. However, the more conservative rules introduce a new risk—a 20 percent chance the study will be needlessly stopped because of a statistically meaningless temporary uptick in the death rate. "You can't ask for a more highly monitored trial than the one we're doing," says its director, Dr. William Hiatt of the University of Colorado. "Just a handful of excess mortality, which could happen by chance, will stop this trial." He and others say the study should go on, because the super-aspirin being tested is better than the ones that failed. It binds more tightly to the platelets and does not fade away as dramatically between doses. But opinions among cardiologists are split over whether the drug is different enough to reasonably expect a better outcome.[1] Don't be fooled when drug companies say that a study is "highly monitored" as if that's what's important. It's not just monitoring we want, but accountability. What we want is assurance that drug trials will be stopped when drugs are found to be dangerous. What we seem to be getting is a tally of those killed and maimed by drugs while drug companies try to tell us that something other than their drugs is at fault. The ongoing battle to launch a "super aspirin" shows us that when hundreds of millions of dollars are at stake accountability is lost. And so the controversy continues. But are we supposed to accept our role as guinea pigs in highly dubious experiments with such puny benefits? Keep this question in mind when we survey the traditional approaches of allopathic medicine in treating arthritis.

However, a dangerous situation is being made even more complicated for the medical consumer. Allopathic medicine and its adherents are not the only ones who can be held responsible for the inadequate range of choices for treating arthritis. Although they have guided the medical consumers' options for many decades, now they have a competitor—the drug companies themselves. And patients are even combining drugs as a result. A new government survey of physicians found that Americans who visited a doctor's office in 1999 were far more likely to receive more than one drug than patients were in 1985. The statistics showed that all ages of patients were increasingly relying on prescription medicines in all classes of drugs, with the notable exception of antibiotics. In 1985 about 61 percent of visits to doctors resulted in patients receiving a medicine or a vaccine. This pattern increased to 66 percent in 1999 but those given prescriptions were much more likely to get multiple drugs, said Catharine W. Burt, chief of the ambulatory care statistics branch at the National Center for Health Statistics, which conducted the survey. The increase in prescribing "is just a lot more than we would have expected just from the aging of the population," Burt said.

But there is a new factor being exploited by the pharmaceutical companies. Drug advertising, especially the promotion of drugs directly to the public, seems to be contributing to the trend. "The ones that are heavily marketed are, in fact, heavily prescribed," Burt said. The survey's findings suggest that direct-to-consumer advertising has made a big impact on sales of medications which are not always the best medications for people to take. Now, the fastest-growing category of health care expenditures is spending for prescription drugs. This new information comes from a survey of a representative national sample of office-based physicians. It shows that medication, usually a prescription, was provided at 501 million of the more than 756 million visits to the doctor that Americans made during 1999. In 1999, 146 drugs were prescribed per 100 visits, a 33 percent increase over the 1985 figure of 109 drugs per 100 visits. Drugs to treat kidney, circulatory, and heart diseases were the top category. But the most frequently prescribed drug, Claritin, is for allergy symptoms. Also among the top 10 were Lipitor, a cholesterol-lowering medicine; Prilosec, a drug for heartburn and for stomach and duodenal ulcers; and Celebrex, a new drug for arthritis. The survey examined the use of 104 drugs approved by the Food and Drug Administration between 1997 and 1999, and found evidence suggesting that marketing was closely related to frequency of prescribing. Drugs that were heavily advertised were much more likely than others to be in the top 20 percent of new drugs prescribed. It found that four new drugs—Celebrex and Vioxx for arthritis, Singulair for asthma and Detrol for overactive bladder—accounted for 12 percent of the estimated $17 billion increase in drug spending that occurred between 1998 and 1999. Nancy M. Ostrove, deputy director of the FDA's division of drug marketing advertising and communication, said, "Manufacturers spend money on promotion to the extent that they believe that there's a good market." Whether advertising causes prescribing or whether increases in both are driven by consumer demand is impossible to say, she added. Burt tried to find a positive aspect within the allopathic paradigm to this dangerous consumer direction by pointing out that antibiotic prescribing declined by 14 percent in 1999 compared with 1985—potentially good news because overprescribing of antibiotics for infections that do not require them has been blamed as a factor in the rise of bacteria resistant to the drugs.[2]

The New York Times reported in May 2001 that retail prescription drug spending in America increased for the fifth straight year in 2000, rising 20% from the previous year and totaling sales of $132 billion. Researchers said more aggressive marketing by drug companies of more expensive drugs contributed to the growth. The top sellers include Vioxx and Celebrex, an arthritis medicine marketed by Pharmacia.[3,4] The revolution in recent communications' technology allowing drug companies speedier access to medical consumers has lead to a diminished role for actual caution and knowledge dispensed by the physician. The lethal threat lurking in this irresponsible situation is illustrated by a recent article in the *New England Journal of Medicine*. It reports that infliximab, an immune-suppressing drug from a class of drugs called anti-TNF (Tumor Necrosis Factor) used to treat rheumatoid arthritis and Crohn's disease, is behind 70 reported cases of tuberculosis (TB) among U.S. patients who received the medication. The cases, at least four of which were fatal, were reported to the Food and Drug Administration between 1998 and May of 2001. Earlier reports in 1995 of indomethacin-treated rats developing TB should have cautioned pharmaceutical companies who continue to make stronger and stronger immune-suppressing drugs.[5] Researchers who reviewed the infliximab TB cases say that the immune-system protein that the drug suppresses—called tumor necrosis factor alpha (TNF-alpha)—appears to be key in controlling TB infection. Since the drug's approval in 1998, nearly 150,000 people worldwide have received infliximab infusions. In August, the Pennsylvania-based Centocor, which markets infliximab as Remicade, announced it was changing the drug's prescribing information to address the TB concerns. The revised labeling will state that patients should be tested and treated for inactive, or latent, TB prior to infliximab therapy. Latent TB refers to a chronic, but symptomless and noncontagious, infection. Such TB infections are prevalent throughout the world because in most people the immune system is able to suppress TB bacteria. Up to 15 million Americans are estimated to have latent TB infections. Latent TB can become active when the immune system is suppressed, as it is in patients on infliximab. Active TB usually attacks the lungs, causing symptoms such as a severe cough, chest pain and weight loss. It is spread through the air from person to person.[6] Such cases as this are cautionary enough for modern consumers, but how much more lethal is it when new drugs are marketed in an environment of hyperpromotional hysteria? A *New York Times* article reports on this hyperpromotional hysteria that has reached illegal heights in marketing Remicade. Centocor is a marketing subsidiary of Johnson & Johnson that

has been telling doctors how they can make extra money by prescribing Remicade, a very expensive treatment for rheumatoid
arthritis. A document available to doctors on Centocor's Web site
was pulled when there were complaints about a document where
doctors could calculate their "estimated revenue per patient" from
prescribing the drug. The "revenue" was the difference between
what Medicare pays doctors for Remicade, which is given intra-
venously in their offices, and the lower amount that Centocor
charged doctors for the drug. The drug is one of the few rheumatoid arthritis treatments that Medicare covers. *The New York
Times* interviewed Dr. Paul April, a rheumatologist in Tulsa, Okla-
homa, who said that other doctors have told him that Centocor
representatives had invited them to meetings where they could
learn about how they could profit from Remicade. He said that
the rheumatology field is now abuzz with discussion of the money
to be made. Dr. April said he believed that some doctors were
prescribing Remicade, which can cost more than $20,000 a year,
before they tried lower-cost generic drugs. *The Times* reports that
sales of Remicade were $658 million last year, more than double
the $256 million in sales in 2000, according to NDCHealth, a
health care information company. According to the federal government, Medicare's payments for Remicade skyrocketed last
year. Medicare paid at least $141 million for Remicade last year—
almost three times the $48 million the government paid for the
drug in 2000.[7]

We'll be talking a lot about the side effects of anti-arthritic
drugs in this chapter but it's becoming clear that these aren't side
effects as much as actual drug effects. It's not a question of
whether side effects occur but what will they be and when will
they happen. Surely the effects that are desired by drug companies and doctors are beneficial effects that alleviate pain and suf-

fering? But do the side effects outweigh the benefits? It cannot be denied any longer that the EFFECTS of these drugs are also very harmful.

ACETAMINOPHEN

Authors in a recent study recommended that the over-the-counter drug acetaminophen be added to the list of medications causing anaphylaxis.[8] Acetaminophen (Tylenol) enjoyed a surge in popularity when the severe side effects of NSAIDs and aspirin became public because PR from pharmaceutical companies promoted it as a safe alternative. However, acetaminophen is not harmless. Perhaps it causes less gastrointestinal bleeding but it has serious side effects such as liver and kidney damage, which may be harder to diagnose initially than gastrointestinal bleeding. It also causes ongoing liver damage, which is often irreparable. It is especially dangerous when given frequently to children under the guise of being safer than aspirin. Even in as little as two days of administering acetaminophen for fever, almost ten percent of young subjects had elevated liver enzymes.[9] Unfortunately, acetaminophen is found in dozens of drugs used for colds, coughs, flu, and headache. It's also very hard on the liver of people who've had hepatitis, and should not be taken if you drink alcohol. Other side effects of acetaminophen include rash, dizziness, open sores, jaundice, fever, hypoglycemic coma, low white blood cell count, easy bruising, and excessive bleeding. And it interacts with many other drugs making it unpredictably dangerous.[10]

Both aspirin and NSAIDs cause gastrointestinal bleeding.[11] The annual death toll due to NSAIDs is about 16,400 and over 100,000 people are hospitalized every year for NSAID complications.[12] One third of patients with side effects due to NSAIDs and aspirin have developed peptic ulcers. A further hazardous interaction occurs when you take NSAIDs or aspirin with alcohol. Your risk of developing gastrointestinal bleeding increases four times. Aspirin not only reduces fever, and relieves pain, but it also reduces inflammation unlike acetaminophen which only works on pain and fever. But there are many side effects including ringing in the ears, allergic reactions, stomach pain, and gastrointestinal bleeding. Aspirin is contraindicated in children and pregnancy due to an association with Reye's syndrome and some forms of asthma. Aspirin interacts with many other medications making it even more dangerous and may aggravate existing liver or kidney damage. (PDR)

IBUPROFEN

The acronym NSAID covers any pain killer that isn't a steroid but the most common NSAID is ibuprofen (Advil). Ibuprofen was approved for use by the FDA in 1974. It is found in over forty medications, some of them available over-the-counter. Ibuprofen is recommended for treatment of both osteoarthritis and rheumatoid arthritis; it reduces inflammation, fever, and is a pain reliever. Because it is no longer patented and has been around for about thirty years it is perceived to be relatively safe to take, but it has a long list of adverse reactions in the PDR. They include: abdominal pain, agranulocytosis, anemia, aplastic anemia, aseptic meningitis, azotemia, blurred vision, bullous rash, confusion, constipation, diarrhea, drowsiness, dyspepsia, dysphagia, edema, elevated hepatic enzymes, esophageal stricture, esophageal ulceration, esophagitis, flatulence, gastritis, GI bleeding, GI performation, headache, hearing loss, heart failure, hematuria, hemolytic anemia, hepatitis, hyperkalemia, hypertension, hyperuricemia, interstitial nephritis, jaundice, maculopapular rash, nausea/vomiting, nephrotic syndrome, neutropenia, odynophagia, pancreatitis, pancytopenia, peptic ulcer, peripheral edema, photophobia, photosensitivity, platelet dynfunction, proteinuria, pseudotumor cerebri, pyrosis (heartburn), renal papillary necrosis, thrombocytopenia, tinnitis, toxic epidermal necrolysis, urticaria, vasculitis, and visual impairment.

In lay terms, package inserts advise you to report to a healthcare professional as soon as possible if you have: signs of bleeding—bruising, pinpoint red spots on the skin, black tarry stools, blood in the urine, unusual tiredness or weakness; signs of an allergic reaction—difficulty breathing or wheezing, skin rash, redness, blistering or peeling skin, hives, or itching, swelling of eyelids, throat, lips; blurred vision; change in the amount of urine passed; chest pain; fast heartbeat; fever, chills, muscle aches and pains; pain or difficulty passing urine; or stomach pain or cramps. The package insert also tells you that a few other side effects that usually do not require medical attention include: diarrhea, dizziness, drowsiness, gas or heartburn, headache, nausea, and vomiting—unless, of course, they become severe! In spite of these long lists they do not include all the possible side effects reports. There have been reports of death by asthma due to ibuprofen;[13] also, "severe generalized reaction" to the drug.[14] And early studies cautioned against taking ibuprofen with heart medication, predicting adverse reactions as well as direct cardio-toxic effects.[15] The way ibuprofen works is not known exactly but it is believed that it inhibits the synthesis and/or the release of prostaglandins. There are prostaglandins that cause inflammation but others that carry out many metabolic functions. The side effects of ibuprofen come when these other prostaglandins are inhibited.

KETOPROFEN

Ketoprofen (Orudis) treats fever, pain, and inflammation but it causes dizziness, rashes, stomach pain, digestive upset, itching and stomach erosion. (PDR)[16] It also causes strong photosensitivity, which means people taking the drug must stay out of the sun or they will develop skin rashes.[17,18] This is especially unfortunate for people who take this drug internally as suppositories or in skin cream form.[19] In one study on guinea pigs all animals tested with ketoprofen developed photosensitivity.[20] The height of arrogance in the testing of drugs such as ketoprofen is evidenced when you see what's really going on in scientific studies. In one instance the subjects were twenty-four healthy, male, Caucasian volunteers who received either oral ketoprofen 100 mg twice daily, or prednisolone 5 mg twice daily, or placebo twice daily for 7.5 days. Blood tests done after the week-long trial indicated no changes in several intricate measures of white blood cells. But if one is not fooled by the intricacy of the testing one would realize that the test is probably utterly worthless because it was done on healthy white males whereas the drugs being tested are usually used on older white females with different forms of arthritis, who use these drugs for more than one week. Merely reading the title of the study might give doctors the impression that ketoprofen does not affect white blood cells, but all it shows is that it didn't affect the white blood cells of a group of young men in a very short period of time.[21]

NAPROXEN

Naproxen (Aleve) is another NSAID that relieves fever, pain, and inflammation but causes the same side effects as all the others:

skin rash, rhinitis, itching, stomach pain, digestive upset, and dizziness. (PDR)[22, 23, 24, 25] Even taking these NSAIDs for a few days can lead to stomach upset for as long as a month with nausea, gas, heartburn, diarrhea, and constipation. And the side effects don't end there. These drugs should only be taken for a few days at a time. But since they are available over-the-counter, people feel it makes them safer to take. Long-term use of NSAIDs, including acetaminophen, can make arthritis worse by inhibiting collagen synthesis and accelerating the destruction of cartilage. They are also destructive to the liver and can cause elevated liver enzymes, jaundice and hepatitis. The kidneys fare no better and you can have urinary frequency, urinary tract infection and kidney dysfunction. With long-term use fatigue, headaches, drowsiness, and nervousness can occur as well as an aggravation of existing depression and psychosis. (PDR) According to the *Physician's Desk Reference* the following symptoms can occur: breast enlargement in men, impotence, menstrual disturbance, blood disorders, hearing disturbances, shortness of breath, blood sugar changes, weight gain or loss, mineral imbalance, and muscle weakness or cramps. Naproxen's affects on the hormones such as impotence and menstrual disturbance are often not attributed to the drug. Men and women with these side effects will accept a prescription for Viagra for impotence, or Sarafem, the new Prozac for premenstrual tension syndrome, before stopping their NSAID.

Drugs themselves cause many side effects but even as the liver is trying to disarm drugs and remove them from the body, intermediary drug metabolites can also cause harm. A study confirming this fact found that metabolites of NSAID naproxen and acetaminophen caused lowering of platelet levels and blood clotting problems.[26] The author of a recent review made an interesting admission that as of 2002 we don't really know whether the various anti-inflammatory drugs for osteoarthritis are actually improving or impairing joint function! Apparently the studies that have been done are contradictory and confusing. Drugs such as sodium salicylate and indomethacin inhibit the synthesis of carti-lage matrix, and indomethacin damaged joint structure, which is exactly what you don't want to happen in treating osteoarthritis. Some drugs such as naproxen and tiaprofenic acid had the oppo-site effects on articular cartilage in different studies.[27] One study assessed the effects of the anti-inflammatory drugs diclofenac, piroxicam, indomethacin, naproxen, nabumetone, nimesulide, and meloxicam on mitochondrial respiration, ATP synthesis, and membrane potential. All but naproxen stimulated basal and uncoupled respiration, inhibited ATP synthesis, and collapsed membrane potential in mitochondria—the basic organ of respira-tion and energy production in the body. Nabumetone inhibited O2 uptake in intact cells and in whole heart culture, whereas the other five drugs stimulated respiration. The study concluded that the sensitive mitochondria are readily targeted by most anti-inflammatory drugs.[28] Another study investigated the very real occurrence of high blood pressure caused by NSAIDs and asked the question, what is the clinical significance? We would think the answer to that question would be to avoid those drugs. A pool-ing of studies on NSAID use and hypertension showed that even in younger adults NSAIDs produced clinically significant increases in blood pressure of 5mm Hg.

Piroxicam, naproxen and indomethacin had the greatest, and sulindac the smallest, hypertensive effect. When data from the elderly was added, those on NSAIDs were seen to have a 40% increased risk of being diagnosed with hypertension and a 1.7 fold higher risk of being prescribed anti-hypertensive drugs compared with non users. The authors remind us that a 5 to 6 mm Hg increase in diastolic blood pressure over several years may be associated with a 67% increase in total stroke risk and a 15% increase in coronary heart disease events. They urged doctors to avoid excessive use of NSAID treatment and look for alternatives.[29]

PIROXICAM

Piroxicam or Feldene is an NSAID that has been implicated in the destruction of healthy chondrocytes (cells that make connective tissue). One study demonstrated that piroxicam inhibited proliferation and synthesis of specific proteins in chondrocytes. And severely-damaged chondrocytes in patients with severe osteoarthritis were even more inhibited. The conclusion was that piroxicam should be used only during a period of joint effusion. One would think the drug would have been banned altogether given that it damages connective tissue.[30] Piroxicam has a host of other side effects including photodermatitis,[31,32,33] bullous dermatosis,[34] and cholestatic hepatitis.[35] When someone has a sensitivity to one NSAID, such as piroxicam, it is becoming clear that there is cross-reactivity to other similar drugs.[36]

An important study followed the funding of NSAID trials and found that when the manufacturer paid for the study, the drug was almost always reported as being equal to or superior in efficacy and toxicity to the comparison drug. The study went on to report that these claims of superiority, especially in regard to side effect profiles, are often not supported by trial data. This study raises concerns about selective publication or biased interpretation of results in manufacturer-associated trials,[37] Anthranilic acid derivatives are a group of nonsteroidal anti-inflammatory drugs that include glafenine and fenamates. Hypersensitivity reactions to these drugs have been documented.[38]

A very real side effect of NSAIDs is getting hooked on other drugs. Many people who take NSAIDs daily do get sensitive stomachs and are put on an anti-acid such as Tagamet to block stomach acid from burning the irritated stomach lining. Without stomach acid, food does not get broken down and minerals don't get acted on by stomach acid to make them absorbable, resulting in malnutrition and nutrient deficiencies. An irritated and inflamed gastrointestinal tract can lead to food allergies which in turn further aggravates arthritic pain, keeping you awake at night. Sleeping pills are added to the mix which makes getting up at night to go to the bathroom a dangerous journey, ending up in thousands of fractured hips. There is an additional concern with the intake of powerful medications such as NSAIDs and that is driving while medicated. Just as we warn people not to drive while drinking there should be similar warnings about driving under the influence of strong medicine. A study reported in the *Journal of Epidemiology* found that older drivers who have heart disease, arthritis, have had a stroke, or are taking certain kinds of medications are more likely to become involved in car crashes. Investigators reviewed the driving records of more than 900 adults over age 65; 426 had been involved in car accidents in 1996. Drivers taking NSAIDs had a 70% increased risk of being involved in an accident. The researchers felt that medications "may not only affect driving performance but also impair judgment and reaction time."[39] This study was only on the over-65 age group and is only the tip of the iceberg adding to the death and disability caused by an overly-medicated society.

CELEBREX

Cox-2 Inhibitors such as Celebrex and Vivox are the latest prescription drugs approved by the FDA for the treatment of arthritic pain and inflammation. They were developed to bypass the gastrointestinal side effects of bleeding and stomach pain. Cycloxygenase (Cox) enzymes Cox-1 and Cox-2 are seen as switches to activate the inflammatory response in cells because they stimulate production of substances in the joints that can cause inflammation and pain. However, they do much more in the body, affecting the kidneys, stomach lining, and blood-clotting factors like platelets. Researchers felt that by inhibiting only the Cox-2 enzymes they could allow the Cox-1 enzymes to continue to protect the kidneys and not interrupt the body's blood clotting factors. But it wasn't long before they found that these new drugs caused negative side effects. Celebrex and Vivox not only caused gastrointestinal problems such as nausea, vomiting, heartburn, indigestion, diarrhea, and abdominal pain but are implicated in studies showing that they double the risk of heart attack.[40]

An editorial in the *British Medical Journal* (BMJ) in 2002 said that research showing that Celebrex had fewer stomach side effects than ibuprofen was flawed. In a study in the September 2000 *Journal of the American Medical Association* (JAMA) patients taking Celebrex did have fewer stomach side effects than those who took NSAIDs. That study looked at 8,000 patients with arthritis, and those on Celebrex had a 52% to 65% lower risk of gastrointestinal problems than did those on either ibuprofen or another NSAID called Cataflam Overall, and 1.4% of patients on those NSAIDs suffered ulcer symptoms compared with less than 1% of those taking Celebrex. But the *BMJ* editorial says the original study contained significant design flaws. It combined findings from two separate studies, and included results from only the first 6 months of data, whereas the studies collected data for a total of 12 and 15 months. When data from the entire study period were analyzed, Celebrex appears to produce as many ulcer complications as the two NSAIDs.[41]

The Washington Post reported on the *BMJ* report. It said that in the summer of 2001, before the Celebrex *JAMA* article was published, it was sent to medical expert Dr. M. Michael Wolfe, a gastroenterologist at Boston University, who was impressed by what he read. Wolfe and a colleague provided a cautiously favorable editorial to accompany it. But in February 2002, when Wolfe was shown the complete data from the same study as a member of the Food and Drug Administration's arthritis advisory committee, he said he saw a different picture. "We were flabbergasted," he said. He didn't realize that the study had lasted a year, not six months. And almost all of the ulcer complications that occurred during the second half of the study were in Celebrex users. Wolfe said, "I am furious . . . I wrote the editorial. I looked like a fool, but . . . all I had available to me was the data presented in the article." *The Washington Post* interviewed *JAMA's* editor, Catherine D. DeAngelis, who said that the journal's editors were not informed about the missing data. She said, "I am disheartened to hear that they had those data at the time that they submitted [the manuscript] to us . . . We are functioning on a level of trust that was, perhaps, broken." The study's 16 authors included faculty members of eight medical schools. All authors were either employees of Pharmacia, Celebrex's manufacturer, or paid consultants of the company.[42] Even the Advisory Panel to the U.S. Food and Drug Administration (FDA), in the beginning stages of acceptance and labeling, advised that Pharmacia, the makers of Celebrex, did not have enough evidence to claim their popular arthritis drug is safer for the stomach than traditional non-steroidal anti-inflammatory drugs (NSAIDs) like ibuprofen. The makers of Celebrex were asking that the warning label for gastrointestinal side effects be dropped. But the FDA said that larger studies were needed before they could drop a warning about gastrointestinal risks that all NSAIDS carry on their packaging. The panel agreed that Pharmacia had not established a "clinically meaningful" safety advantage over NSAIDs and that data from the CLASS study would not support a superiority claim. What was disturbing to the FDA panel was that although the trial showed a decrease in gastrointestinal complications that was twice that of other drugs, this trend was reversed among subjects who also took low-dose aspirin. Since many older people take low-dose aspirin daily to protect against heart attack, this constituted a great risk. The panel also did not feel that Celebrex was safe for people with existing ulcers. But the panel did not ask for new labeling to protect people on aspirin or with existing ulcers.[43]

The interaction between Celebrex and aspirin was already known. In a *JAMA* study in September 2000, patients taking Celebrex and daily aspirin had a 450% increase in GI complications. For patients taking NSAIDs, daily aspirin use raised the risks up to 335%. And, "No difference was noted in the incidence of cardiovascular events between celecoxib and NSAIDs, irrespective of aspirin use."[44]

With all these side effects from arthritic drugs one would imagine that medical doctors and organizations like the Arthritis Foundation would try to find safer alternatives. However, they have a very suspicious view of non-drug treatments. The Arthritis Foundation admits that one of the most common questions that people with arthritis ask is whether diet can affect them. They say that research is being done to define the role of diet in arthritis and that there are some scientific reasons why food may have an effect. But they do agree that excessive weight affects the joints. They don't endorse any specific diet for arthritis but recommend that everyone eat a balanced diet that includes a variety of foods: plenty of vegetables, fruits and whole-grain products. Instead of eliminating sugar and saturated fat they suggest taking it in moderation. About vitamins and minerals they just say to take the RDA (Recommended Daily Allowance), which only staves off vitamin and mineral deficiencies. The Arthritis Foundation suggests that double blind studies on food intake in arthritic patients and controls needs to be done to "prove" what foods do and do not help this condition.

The Arthritis Foundation's "Guide to Alternative Therapies" mostly instructs its readers to avoid alternatives. It begins by suggesting that a joyless painful life of disability may make you vulnerable to seek out alternatives.

Exactly. Written in 2000, it says that 43 million people with arthritis are looking for alternative therapies and that half of Americans are already trying unconventional ones. It seems that the Arthritis Foundation doesn't want you to do anything unconventional. It allows that meditation might help your stress, anxiety and pain. Or that yoga and acupuncture, preferably done at a local hospital or HMO, will offer you some relief but reminds you that most alternative therapies are useless at best and some are dangerous. The article then goes on to denounce hucksters with miracle cures, dietary supplements that vary in effectiveness, quality and safety that not only take your money and raise false hopes but are harmful because they keep you from using proven therapies. They are saying that not taking proven drug therapies can be dangerous!

* * *

The Arthritis Foundation drums in this message, "Don't expect a 'cure' from complementary therapies." They say: "We can't repeat this enough: There is no cure for most kinds of arthritis." Even that is not enough advice because they know people are going to try alternatives, so they list "Seven Danger Signs About A Therapist"—a list that could be just as readily applied to your medical doctor:

1. "Promises you can be 'cured.' Many therapies may help your condition, but there is no cure for most kinds of arthritis and related diseases—and no reputable practitioner will promise a cure." So, you are warned away from anyone who says they can help you. It's a catch-22. And if you do break away from the bonds of allopathic medicine and are "cured" by an alternative medicine practitioner, your arthritis specialist will say that the original diagnosis was wrong. After all, arthritis is incurable!

2. "Tells you to stop or decrease prescription medications. Never stop or change doses of prescription drugs without talking to your physician." It is sound advice to never abruptly stop your prescription. But this advice relegates patients to forever taking powerful medication instead of finding less harmful non-drug solutions.

3. "Advises a severely restricted diet. No, we don't mean a vegetarian diet—we mean a diet that is extreme or involves eliminating many types of foods." The best dietary advice for arthritis is to avoid sugar, wheat, dairy, caffeine and alcohol, but these suggestions would be considered "extreme" by the Arthritis Foundation.

4. "Insists you pay in advance for a series of expensive treatments. No practitioner can predict how you might respond

to a treatment, and you should not have to pay for treatments you do not receive or need." However, health care insurance is paid for in advance, and inability to pay often closes hospital doors and doctors' doors.

5. "Cannot show you a license or a certificate from an approved school or organization in his or her specialty. Anyone can claim to be an 'expert'." An approved school or organization in the eyes of the Arthritis Foundation is usually one that promotes drugs and surgery.

6. "Advises you to keep the treatment a secret from your doctor, or anyone else."

   Many doctors will "fire" a patient for taking alternative treatments and often patients make the decision not to upset their doctor by talking about alternative medicine treatments.

7. "Suggests or asks for an intimate sexual relationship." This is an incredible citation in a list of tips on choosing alternative therapists. By including it in this list it infers and implies that alternative therapists might also be sexual perverts.

The Arthritis Foundation also has a helpful guide called "What's the Alternative?" in their Arthritis Today publication, which basically cautions and chastises the 65 percent of the readers who have taken a dietary supplement in the past six months. They don't remind readers that every metabolic function in the body depends on vitamins and minerals. Rather they sarcastically say, "No doubt, people with arthritis are helping to make supplements a thriving industry." They admit that it must be difficult for people to separate the wheat from the chaff and recommend their "2002-2003 Supplement Guide" to help make the important decision about whether to take a supplement or not.

A select panel of experts, all medical doctors, and one Registered Dietitian, from universities and hospitals "scrutinized the most current, comprehensive and well-respected supplement and herb books and databases; interviewed top researchers at supplement companies, universities and other institutions; and reviewed and distilled the most current scientific research." There were no Naturopathic Doctors, Clinical Nutritionists, Osteopaths, Herbalists, Homeopaths on their panel. While doctors warn patients not to turn to alternatives they give very little hope that their research will find a cure in the near future. In answer to a frequently asked question, "When will research find a cure for arthritis?" they reply, "Because medical science has the ability to cure problems as diverse as appendicitis and ear infections, we have come to expect that any disease can be cured. Frankly, and unfortunately, however, most forms of arthritis and related diseases are not among those considered curable." Wanting to give people some hope they say, "But the news isn't all bad. Research into arthritis treatment has paid off. Thanks to advances in research, doctors have more drugs at their disposal . . . and doctors can diagnose diseases at the earliest and most treatable stages."

DISEASE-MODIFYING ANTI-RHEUMATIC DRUGS (DMARDS)

Let's look at one of the latest rheumatoid arthritis drugs as an example of the direction modern medicine is taking in the approach to this disease. In November 2001, Amgen, an independent biotech company produced a new rheumatoid arthritis drug called Kineret. It's only available by subcutaneous injection. Kineret is a biological response modifier, called a disease-modifying anti-rheumatic drug (DMARD). It is genetically-engineered from an intestinal organism called E. Coli. The drug manages the signs and symptoms of rheumatoid arthritis by blocking the biological protein Interleukin-1, which builds up in joints causing pain, swelling, and stiffness.[45] We aren't told what other things Interleukin-1 is responsible for but we get some idea that Interleukin-1 is necessary to fight infections when we look at the list of side effects. Kineret should not be used if you have an infection that requires antibiotics. This presents an interesting conundrum because some researchers and doctors feel that arthritis may, in fact, be caused by infection.[46,47,48,49,50] So, if most people with rheumatoid arthritis already have infection, by taking Kineret—which reduces their body's ability to fight infection—they could have a real problem.

Asthma is also a contraindication for taking this drug because it can lead to infection. We are also told that you cannot use Kineret if you have an allergy to proteins made from the bacterial cells of E. Coli, from which the drug originates. The immediate question is, how can you know that? As part of its immune suppressing action Kineret also decreases the number of a type of white blood cell, which means you have to take blood tests every three months while on the drug and for up to a year after getting off it. But taking blood tests doesn't protect you from getting this side effect. It just lets your doctor know that you're in trouble. Other adverse reactions include abdominal pain, antibody formation against the drug in one quarter of patients, diarrhea, bruising, edema, redness, headache, injection site rejection, and sinusitis. (PDR) Interestingly, Amgen is marketing the drug to about 300,000 patients with moderate to severe rheumatoid arthritis who have failed traditional treatments, but one of the contraindications is kidney damage, which is a common side effect of most rheumatoid arthritis drugs. So, many people who have failed other drug treatments could already have kidney damage which sets them up for more side effects with Kinerat. The approval for Kinerat was based on the use of the drug in 2,600 patients.

The results were that after 6 months of therapy, 38 percent of Kineret patients as compared to 22 percent of patients taking placebo achieved a 20 percent improvement in symptoms, according to American College of Rheumatology criteria. That means there was only a 16 percent difference in the drug group and the group that got nothing. And if your pain was at a level of 5, on a scale of one to 5 with 5 being severe, now your pain is at a level of 4. You have to wonder if the side effects warrant such a minimal result.[51]

Next comes the cost. The company, Amgen, told the Associated Press that the cost of the drug was about $11,088 per year.[52] But Centrus, an "independent pharmacy benefits management company," warns that Kineret's prefilled syringe is $61.57 which adds up to $1,847 a month and $22,164 a year.[53] Most of this information is readily available on the Kineret website under a heading called "The Advantage of New Scientific Thinking." But what about commonsense thinking and practical thinking? Apparently there is no thinking about any alternative therapies for arthritis beyond expensive drugs and surgery.

ROFECOXIB

Rofecoxib or Vioxx by Merck, approved by the FDA in May 1999, is another COX-2 inhibitor that came along shortly after Celebrex was released by Pharmaceia in December 1998. It's used for mild to moderate pain of arthritis or for painful periods. Doctors who prescribe this medication should not give it to patients who have allergic reactions to aspirin, other salicylates, other NSAIDs, foods, dyes or preservatives; patients with anemia, asthma; cigarette smokers; dehydrated patients; those who drink more than 3 alcohol-containing beverages a day; patients with heart or circulation problems such as heart failure or leg edema; patients with high blood pressure, kidney disease, liver disease, nasal polyps, stomach bleeding or ulcers, taking blood thinners, taking hormones such as prednisone (steroids); or patients who are pregnant or trying to get pregnant, or breast-feeding. In clinical trials rofecoxib shows an efficacy that compares to the much older NSAIDs, ibuprofen and diclofenac, in patients with osteoarthritis. So the question arises, do we need yet another anti-inflammatory drug? The answer from the drug companies may be that ibuprofen is no longer patented so it can be made much cheaper in a competitive market. Whereas a new patent on a new anti-inflammatory allows the drug company to charge higher prices. Vioxx was also heavily marketed, as was Celebrex, as a drug that would not cause gastrointestinal (GI) bleeding. However, that is not the case. A study called the Vioxx GI Outcomes Research (VIGOR) showed that in patients treated with rofecoxib 50 mg/day, the risk of GI toxicity is less than with naproxen 1000 mg/day.[54] However, the VIGOR study demonstrated an increased risk of cardiovascular thrombotic events with rofecoxib as compared to naproxen.[55] What you avoid in GI toxicity you make up for in heart problems.

Another side effect, aseptic meningitis, began to develop in people taking Vioxx. There were seven patients who developed meningitis reported between May 1999, when it was approved, to February 2001. Their symptoms began within 1 to 12 days after starting the drug. These included headache, fever, sensitivity to light, neck stiffness and confusion. Further confirmation of the Vioxx connection was that one patient was restarted on Vioxx twice, and both times the symptoms of meningitis reappeared.

And these were not all elderly, debilitated patients. They ranged in age from 16 to 67.[56] The journal Science reports that research in mice suggests that COX-2 inhibitors, such as Celebrex and Vioxx, could trigger a chain of events potentially harmful to the cardiovascular system. This could explain why a recent major drug trial on Vioxx showed higher rates of heart attacks and heart disease in patients compared with naproxen. Researchers say that COX-2 inhibitors could create an imbalance that promotes blood clotting and blood vessel constriction. COX-2 is required to prevent platelets from clumping and to promote blood vessel dilation. Drug companies hoped that COX-2 drugs would just inhibit inflammation but they don't operate in a vacuum and are not allowed to do their normal work of preventing platelets from clumping. As if it would make a great difference in prescribing habits of doctors already conditioned to think that the COX-2 inhibitors are safer than NSAIDs, Merck & Co. Inc., the maker of Vioxx, announced that the arthritis drug's labeling would be changed to state that it carries higher cardiovascular risks than naproxen. This labeling change was required by the FDA following the Vioxx-naproxen trial.[57]

The spin given to DMARDs is that they relieve symptoms and help to control rheumatoid arthritis by modifying the actual disease process. They still don't treat the disease or cure the disease but still just relieve symptoms by insinuating themselves into what scientists believe is the disease process. Given that we still don't know exactly how rheumatoid arthritis or osteoarthritis are created, it is interesting that scientists still feel confident in disrupting what they think is the disease process. And they do this with drugs that are so toxic that they are used in severe forms of cancer.

METHOTREXATE

Methotrexate is a cancer drug that has been given a new life as one of the most widely prescribed DMARDs. But because of methotrexate's potential to cause serious side effects, doctors carefully monitor patients who are taking the drug with blood tests. They don't ban the drug from use even though it is so dreadfully toxic. They just take blood tests, which may give patients some sense of security about taking the drug, but blood testing does absolutely nothing about the side effects. Methotrexate is so toxic that it is only taken once a week as a pill, liquid, or injection. While it is given to suppress inflammation, its other effects are to cause abnormalities of bone marrow and liver function.[58] It's off limits to pregnant and nursing women, people using alchool, and people with AIDS or other immune system suppression. Being an auto-immune disease one would think that rheumatoid arthritis patients already have immune system suppression but instead they are the so-called beneficiaries of this very toxic drug. One result of immune suppression is an increase in the incidence of cancer in patients taking methotrexate.[59] Additional side effects of methotrexate may include fatigue, flu-like symptoms, upset stomach, headaches, and mouth sores.

Rheumatoid nodules, which are supposed to be suppressed by methotrexate, may instead be induced by this toxic drug.[60] And the rare disease pneumocystis carinii pneumonia has been induced in rheumatoid arthritic patients with this drug.[61] Another negative effect on the lung includes the condition called pneumonitis as a complication of methotrexate therapy.[62]

Some researchers are getting the idea that vitamin supplements may be beneficial for people with arthritis but they are using them to take the sting out of arthritic drugs such as methotrexate. A

2001 study showed that patients taking folic acid or folinic acid supplements along with the arthritis drug methotrexate had lower rates of liver impairment than those taking just methotrexate. The benefits, according to researchers, were that patients taking the folate supplements were able to continue their drug therapy for longer periods because about 30% of patients discontinue therapy because of toxicity. There was no change in methotrexate's other side effects, such as nausea, dizziness, diarrhea, and fatigue. According to researchers, after 48 weeks, 38% of patients taking the placebo had stopped treatment with methotrexate, compared with 17% of patients taking folic acid and 12% of patients taking folinic acid. Patients taking the placebo had higher levels of liver enzymes indicating liver toxicity than patients taking folate supplements. Of great interest, however, is that by the end of the study, patients taking folate needed higher amounts of methotrexate to achieve the same impact on their arthritis as patients taking methotrexate with placebo.[63] The researchers don't seem to realize that perhaps folate helps to diminish the toxicity of methotrexate by helping to eliminate it from the body and probably the increased doses of methotrexate given to counteract the folate will just build up and cause the same toxicity in the first place.

LEFLUNOMIDE

Leflunomide, called Arava by Avantis pharmaceutical company, is another powerful DMARD that is used in the treatment of rheumatoid arthritis. It is powerful, not in the sense that it can cure rheumatoid arthritis, but because it has strong negative effects on the body. Regular blood tests, including liver function tests and blood counts, are required to monitor patients using leflunomide. Its side effects include gastrointestinal symptoms, skin rashes, and reversible hair loss. It should not be taken by people with active infections, but as we queried earlier, what if rheumatoid arthritis is itself an infectious disease? Because studies have shown that leflunomide can cause birth defects in animals, women of childbearing age must not get pregnant while on the drug.

This warning also applies to men who are planning to father a child. They must make sure the medication is clear from their body when attempting to conceive. One study investigating the mechanism of action found that it suppresses certain inflammatory proteins by genetic interference. No mention was made of measuring its effects on the other thousands of proteins in the body, which are all exposed to such a drug.[64]

Another study showed that leflunomide inhibits DNA synthesis, which is probably not going to be isolated to only inflammatory cells.[65] The not-for profit group Public Citizen lead by Dr. Sidney Wolfe in March of 2002 demanded that the FDA ban leflunomide. They said since it came on the market in 1998 it has been linked to 130 cases of severe liver problems including 12 deaths. Two of those who died were in their 20s. Dr. Wolfe said, "When there are other treatments that are more effective and don't endanger patients as much as this drug, there is absolutely no reason for the FDA to keep Arava on the market." Arava has also been associated with 12 cases of the life-threatening autoimmune disease, Stevens-Johnson Syndrome. Even packaging inserts warn that byproducts of the drug can remain in the body for months, which means that if a reaction is noticed, stopping the drug will not necessarily stop the side effects. Even a recently retired member of the FDA's Arthritis Drugs Advisory Committee, Dr. David E. Yocum, director of the Arizona Arthritis Center at Arizona Health Sciences Center, agrees that the drug should be withdrawn from the market. He said, "I do not believe that the general rheumatologist understands or has any knowledge about these serious and potentially life-threatening complications. I also agree that providing a black box warning concerning these issues may not be effective since no one can predict who will suffer from these complications." "Before it was approved by the FDA, there was evidence that leflunomide led to liver complications, and now the dangers are even clearer," Wolfe said. "No more patients should be subjected to these risks."[66]

Such is the case with so many drugs that reach the marketplace: They are shown to be toxic in preliminary trials, which are often on young, healthy, male subjects on no other medications. But thrown into a sick population often taking several other medications with severe inflammatory conditions, these drugs become monsters. They are let loose and it takes years of lobbying and a mounting body count to get them off the market. By the time they are banned another dozen even more powerful and dangerous drugs have taken their place.

SULFASALAZINE

Sulfasalazine is a combination drug that contains a sulfa drug and an anti-inflammatory and acts as both an antibiotic and to suppress inflammation in people with arthritis. People who are allergic to medications that contain sulfa cannot take sulfasalazine. Its side effects can affect the liver as well as lower the counts of white blood cells and platelets. So, blood monitoring by a physician is required when taking this drug. Other symptoms from taking sulfasalazine may include headaches, upset stomach and rashes. There is even a syndrome named after the drug called the "3-week sulphasalazine syndrome," a rare, but often fatal, immuno-allergic reaction to the drug where patients develop dermatitis, fever, lymphadenopathy, fulminant drug-induced hepatitis leading to multi-organ failure, sepsis and death.[67] And there are reported cases of neurological deterioration, encephalopathy, and toxic hepatitis with the drug.[68]

AZATHIOPRINE

Azathioprine is an immunosuppressant, which means it can prevent the ability of the immune system to respond to an immune challenge. It is given to patients with rheumatoid arthritis to suppress the immune system component of the illness in which the body attacks its own joints. In alternative medicine we know that it is partly the body attacking toxins in the joints that are the real trigger to rheumatoid arthritis and it is the toxins that should be eliminated. Patients using azathioprine must be closely monitored by their doctor for the drug's potential effects on their bone marrow and liver. Other side effects to consider include an increased risk of infection because the patient's own immune system is being intentionally suppressed. Another rare side effect is a severe allergic or hypersensitivity reaction, often consisting of fever, hypotension, and decreased urination. In such cases the correct diagnosis is often missed. The patient is thought to have an infection. Usually all drugs are stopped and a work up for infection begins. When nothing is found the azathioprine is resumed and the allergic reaction is even more pronounced with fever, nausea and vomiting, diarrhea, hypotension, tachycardia and lack of urination, and may lead to liver or kidney damage.[69] A report on the effects of immunosuppressive therapy with prednisolone (with or without azathioprine) on patients with chronic hepatitis showed an increase in activity of the hepatitis[70] and a reactivation of the hepatitis virus in a group of children on immunosuppressive drug therapy.[71]

CYCLOSPORINE

Cyclosporine is another immunosuppressive drug that is often prescribed in combination with methotrexate for treating active, severe rheumatoid arthritis. Cyclosporine's negative effects are on the kidneys, so doctors prescribing the drug must closely monitor patients' blood pressure, kidney function, as well as taking frequent blood tests. But nothing can protect a patient from a fatal anaphalactic reaction after their first treatment.[72]

HYDROXYCHLOROQUINE

Hydroxychloroquine is an anti-malaria drug that has been used to treat rheumatoid arthritis because it relieves swelling, inflammation and pain. Although hydroxychloroquine is sometimes called the safest of the DMARDs, patients taking the drug require regular eye exams to check for retinal damage that hydroxychloroquine can cause. The *PDR* refers to the incidence of this retinal damage as rare, but when it occurs in YOUR eyes, the incidence is 100%! A case of contact dermatitis was diagnosed in a pharmaceutical industry worker on exposure to hydroxychloroquine. After removal from the workplace for four months, re-exposure resulted in dermatitis and asthma. Symptoms only improved after many months and complete removal from exposure.[73]

D-PENCILLAMINE

D-pencillamine is a DMARD that was used in the past but its effects were so horrific that it has fallen out of favor in view of the new drugs being marketed. Or perhaps its patent ran out. D-pencillamine is taken as a pill on an empty stomach, and its usage, as with all the DMARDs, requires close supervision by a physician.

In 1993 a study was done to determine which antirheumatic drugs are discontinued due to side effects. A series of 245 recently diagnosed rheumatoid arthritis patients were followed. Chrysotherapy (gold injections) were often stopped because of toxicity. In older patients sulfasalazine seemed to carry more toxicity than in younger patients. In patients with active disease, initially hydroxychloroquine, sulfasalazine and penicillamine were not as beneficial and were discontinued.[74]

A review of the literature on the treatment of rheumatoid arthritis showed an increase in the use of two or more disease modifying anti-rheumatic drugs. Presumably when doctors find that one drug doesn't work, instead of looking elsewhere for alternatives, they routinely combine two or more drugs in an attempt to knock out the immune system and stop the inflammation in rheumatoid arthritis. In this review the authors found 18 well-conducted, randomized controlled trials using combinations of DMARDs. The 18 trials involved 2,221 patients with only two trials reporting strongly positive results. Six reported moderately positive results and ten gave negative results. Instead of stopping there and saying that the odds for favorable results were two to eighteen, which are very poor odds, the reviewers went on to suggest that a combination of methotrexate, sulfasalazine, and hydroxychloroquine appeared to be effective with an acceptable level of adverse effects.[75] Another review suggested adding corticosteroids to the above three-drug combination to help with side effects due to the drugs.[76] But we are also aware of the long-term adrenal suppression, bone thinning, gastrointestinal bleeding, and immune suppression from the use of corticosteroids.

CORTICOSTEROIDS

The final class of drugs used for arthritis are glucocorticoids. Decades ago they were thought to be a panacea for arthritis sufferers until their side effects surfaced.

Prednisone is the most commonly-prescribed oral corticosteroid. It is classified as an anti-inflammatory, a biological response modifier, an immunosuppressant, and a musculoskeletal agent. Prednisone is about four times more potent than the body's own glucocorticoids. Prednisone, a synthetic form of the body's own natural glucocorticoids was first approved as a drug by the FDA in 1955. Glucocorticoids are hormones naturally produced by the adrenal glands and involved with dozens of metabolic functions. The synthetic drug in high doses can suppress inflammation and immunity so it was immediately put to work to suppress the inflammation of arthritis and block allergic reactions.

It wasn't long before damaging side effects surfaced. One of the most lethal is suppression of the body's own glucocorticoid production called hypothalamic-pituitary-adrenal (HPA) suppression—because the body thinks there is enough, it stops producing its own. Then when the drug is stopped, especially if stopped abruptly, the body goes into severe depletion with none being produced. So, an absolute contraindication in prednisone use is the abrupt discontinuation of the medication; one must be weaned off slowly to allow the body's own production to come back. Other absolute contraindications include: Cushing's syndrome, which is a disease caused by an excess of cortisol production or by excessive use of cortisol or other similar steroid (glucocorticoid) hormones; measles infection, chickenpox, and fungal infection. Otherwise, contraindications include: blood clotting problems, breast feeding, cataracts, children, diabetes, diverticulitis, GI disease, glaucoma, heart failure, hepatic disease, herpes infection, hypertension, hypothyroidism, infection, inflammatory bowel disease, myasthenia gravis, myocardial infarction, osteoporosis, peptic ulcer disease, psychosis, renal disease, seizure disorder, surgery, thromboembolic disease, tuberculosis, ulcerative colitis, vaccination, viral infection, and visual disturbance. (PDR)

PREDNISONE

The descriptions of the adverse reactions or side effects from prednisone use could take up a whole book. They include: abdominal pain, acne vulgaris, adrenocortical insufficiency, amenorrhea, angioedema, anorexia, anxiety, appetite stimulation arthralgia, avascular necrosis, bone fractures, cataracts, constipation, Cushing's syndrome, depression, diabetes, diaphoresis, diarrhea, dysmenorrhea, ecchymosis (bruising), edema, EEG changes, emotional lability, erythema, esophageal ulceration, euphoria, exfoliative dermatitis, exopthalmos, fever, fluid retention, gastritis, glossitis, growth inhibition, headache, heart failure, hirsutism, hypercholesterolemia, hyperglycemia, hypernatremia, hypertension, hypocalcemia, hypokalemia, hypotension, immunosuppression, impaired wound healing, increased intracranial pressure, infection, insomnia, lethargy, menstrual irregularity, metabolic alkalosis, myalgia, myopathy, nausea/vomiting, ocular hypertension, optic neuritis, osteoporosis, palpitations, pancreatitis, papilledema, peptic ulcer, peripheral neuropathy, petechiae, phlebitis, physiological dependence, pseudotumor cerebri, psychosis, restlessness, retinopathy, seizures, sinus tachycardia, skin atrophy, sodium retention, stomatitis, striae, thromboembolism, thrombosis, urinary incontinence, urinary urgency, urticaria, vertigo, visual impairment, weakness, weight gain, weight loss, and withdrawal. (*PDR*) Prednisone interacts with a long list of drug groups comprising hundreds of medications that cause many negative side effects. These include: anticoagulants, antidiabetic drugs, antineoplastic drugs, antithyroid drugs, barbituates, cholinesterase inhibitors, diuretics, estrogens, immunosuppressives, neuromuscular blockers, nonsteroidal anti-inflammatory drugs (NSAIDs), photosensitizing drugs, salicylates, thyroid hormones, toxoids, and vaccines. And the following individual drugs also pose dangers when used with prednisone: amphotericin B, bosentan, digoxin, dofetilide, ephedra, infliximab, isoproterenol, L-asparaginase, Mifepristone-RU-486, Nevirapine, pegaspargase, phenytoin, rifabutin, rifampin, and ritonavir. (*PDR*) In spite of over one hundred contraindications and side effects of prednisone, more reports keep coming in about new adverse reactions. A report in the *International Journal of Dermatology* links multiple dermatofibromas to prednisone.[77]

A recent review article on these steroid drugs gives a long list of negative side effects. Pharmacological doses of glucocorticosteroids given chronically are associated with a variety of negative side effects. They have catabolic effects on protein causing protein wasting and resulting in poor tissue healing. They increase the incidence of infections.[78] They also accelerate bone loss and cause osteoporosis in bones that are already weakened by arthritis.[79,80,81] Corticosteroids create osteoporosis and bone loss by a variety of mechanisms. They reduce intestinal calcium absorption and increase renal calcium excretion. They inhibit osteoblast (bone making) function as well as inhibiting the favorable effects of growth factors and sex hormones on bone. It has recently been recognized that the expression of Vitamin D hormone receptors (VDRs) is suppressed by these medications and that corticosteroids probably induce VDR disorders. Not only the bones are affected but muscle strength also suffers from the use of corticosteroids.[82] Insulin resistance to both liver and peripheral tissue is common with corticosteroid use and may result in diabetes.[83] One of the predictors of a bad outcome in some forms of arthritis is the use of glucocorticoids.[84]

After listing medications as the first line of treatment for arthritis most medical advice moves on to other more benign palliative offerings. These treatments are obviously interspersed with drug therapy but drugs are always at the top of the list of therapies for arthritis. Patients are advised to exercise their joints gently to keep them mobile and to try and build up muscle strength. If they are experience pain or become fatigued they are told to rest. Diet advice is usually a blanket statement to eat with well-balanced diet with no specific advice other than to lose weight if the patient is overweight. Devices such as splints, braces, canes and shoe inserts are described as part of an arthritis management program. Heat and cold therapies to reduce pain and inflammation under the guidance of the doctor are recommended. They include paraffin wax, ultrasound, or moist heat to increase blood circulation and flexibility. Cold packs, cooling sprays, and ointments are recommended to numb the nerves around painful joints.

SURGERY

When all else fails, patients are offered surgery. Diagnostic procedures that involve surgery such as arthroscopy, which offers a fiberoptic view of joints, in some hospitals are associated with an infection rate of 2 percent.[85] In both rheumatoid arthritis and osteoarthritis, damaged joints may be repaired or removed, bones may be fused for more stability, or a patient may have total joint replacement with an artificial joint. In some of the most radical surgical procedures as few as one third of patients experience "good" results.[86] There are a series of problems with such invasive surgery. For example, researchers find that the continuation of the inflammatory process around the hip replacement may lead to loosening of the newly placed hip.[87] And repeat surgery is sometimes indicated.[88] In a group of patients undergoing knee replacement psychological support made a big difference in outcome.[89] Side effects from joint surgery include infections that form around fragments of the joint material or on the prosthesis itself.[90,91,92,93,94,95] Finding accurate methods of detecting infection in and around a joint prosthesis are a source of ongoing research. Allergic reactions or hypersensitivity to prosthesis components also occur.[96,97,98] Even the plaster of paris casting material used to splint or cast a limb after surgery can cause allergic reactions.[99]

CONCLUSION

The remarkable studies presented in this chapter really bring home the point that there has to be a better way to take back our health and to prevent illness in the first place. Any thoughts of there being a magic bullet will have evaporated after reading these pages. One criticism of alternative medicine and natural approaches is that they give patients "false hope" but what could be more false than paying $20,000 per year for a treatment that MIGHT help you improve your symptoms by 20%? Alternative medicine is also called quackery. But one definition of a quack is someone who pretends to be a medic who charges outrageous fees and through promotion and advertising gives the illusion of offering a cure. It seems like the current trend to advertise expensive drugs on television with the promise of a cure fits the definition of quackery to a T. So, I urge you not to be drawn in by the advertising hype surrounding medicine and the promise of a magic bullet. And we offer you in Chapter Four dozens of proven remedies and therapies to help turn your health around and keep you well.

4

ALTERNATIVE THERAPIES

As we have shown in Chapter 3, medical treatments for arthritis fail to cure or even alleviate the disease. For all the thousands of dollars spent on research to find the "cure" for arthritis at least one study reports that rheumatoid arthritis patients are not benefiting from this research and living longer. A group from the Mayo clinic compared the life span of patients with rheumatoid arthritis to those without the disease and found that rheumatoid arthritis patients had a 38% greater risk of death. Those patients with newly diagnosed rheumatoid arthritis had a greater risk of death. Looking at women with rheumatoid arthritis, their risk is even more striking with a 55% increased risk compared to the general population.[1] Such statistics should make people realize that something is not working and it's time for a change, especially since the numbers of people getting arthritis, both rheumatoid arthritis and osteoarthritis, are increasing as the population ages.

WHO GETS ARTHRITIS?

According to the *Morbidity and Mortality Weekly Report* from the CDC (Centers for Disease Control and Prevention) of May 2001, an estimated 43.1 million Americans of all ages report having arthritis. Of that number an estimated 7.8 million report that arthritis limits their daily activities in some way. The data, from 1997, also indicate that the number of people with arthritis has increased by 750,000 people per year since 1990, and the CDC predicts that by 2020, 116 million Americans will be limited by arthritis.[2]

But even a year later more people are reporting arthritis and chronic joint problems. They affect close to 33 percent of American adults; that's about 80 million people, according to a self-reported survey. The survey was carried out by random-digit telephone calls. Surveyors asked participants questions relating to symptoms, pain intensity and diagnosis of arthritis and joint problems. Results indicated that prevalence increased with age, overweight or obesity, physical inactivity and in those who had not completed high school. Women had the highest incidence, and non-Hispanic whites and non-Hispanic blacks had a higher prevalence than those in other ethnic groups.[3]

A recent study found that knee injuries, not regular exercise, sets the stage for knee osteoarthritis. This is important because many people avoid any physical activity once they feel a twinge in their knees. But lack of exercise has its own harmful side effects with muscle wasting and atrophy possibly creating unstable knees. The researchers studied 216 patients who reported onset of arthritis after age 40, with knee pain, swelling or stiffness. Each person in this group was matched to four people without the condition. They found that having a previous knee injury was the only factor that strongly influenced the risk of knee arthritis. People with previous injuries had an eight-times greater risk of knee osteoarthritis, compared with those with no prior knee injuries.[4]

A paper on the epidemiology of rheumatoid arthritis in 2002 found that, instead of occurring in a mostly younger female population aged twenty to fifty, older people are being diagnosed. It lists the risk factors as: genetic, a difficult pregnancy, smoking, obesity, and recent infections.[5] To that list we would add stress, dietary deficiencies, sports injuries and surgery, allergies and chemical sensitivities, pollution and metal toxicity, exposure to harmful chemicals, hormonal imbalance, metabolic problems, and immune system dysfunction. And arthritis is occurring in older people as they accumulate the strains and stresses of a toxic lifestyle.

Coffee drinking, for example, carried a risk of 2.20 in people who drank four or more cups of coffee a day compared to those drinking less.[6] But don't just switch to decaf. Decaffeinated coffee consumption was found to be another risk factor that you can modify. Researchers followed more than 31,000 women aged 55 to 69 included in the Iowa Women's Health Study from 1986 through 1997. A group of 158 women developed rheumatoid arthritis during that time period. They were compared with women who did not develop the disease. It became clear that women drinking four or more cups a day of decaffeinated coffee were at more than twice the risk of developing rheumatoid arthritis. In another similar study, researchers evaluated risk factors for developing rheumatoid arthritis among 64,000 black women followed since 1995 as part of the Black Women's Health Study. Their data showed that drinking more than one cup a day of decaffeinated coffee seemed to quadruple the risk of developing rheumatoid arthritis. The researchers speculate that the use of industrial solvents in the decaffeination process may play a role. This study adds to the evidence that environmental factors play an important role in the development of rheumatoid arthritis.[7]

Another group found that tobacco smoking is a risk factor of rheumatoid arthritis. They also found that low levels of formal education, body mass index, marital or employment status were not significantly associated with risk of rheumatoid arthritis, but that smoking in men was identified as an independent risk factor for the disease.[8]

The role of toxicity in the environment is evidenced in a *Journal of Epidemiology* report. Researchers studied an arthritis-like condition called undifferentiated connective tissue disease (UCTD) that occurs in women with medical implants. The disease is five times more likely in women with non-silicone devices and three times more likely to occur in women with silicone-containing implants compared to women with no implants. UCTD causes pain and swelling in the joints and cold sensitivity, and can be misdiagnosed as arthritis.[9] Many people use hair dyes, which are partially absorbed into the body. A recent study shows that hair dyes used for more than 20 years may cause double the risk of developing rheumatoid arthritis.[10]

Medical research continues to look for the drug that will "cure" rheumatoid arthritis. Gene researchers have suggested that rheumatoid arthritis is a genetic disease and if they could find that gene they could modify it and cure the condition. However, according to a study in the *British Medical Journal* genes may play a small role in rheumatoid arthritis. A study was undertaken of 13 identical and 36 fraternal (non-identical) twin pairs in which at least one twin had rheumatoid arthritis. Interestingly enough in two of the fraternal twin pairs both twins were affected, but in none of the identical twin pairs were both affected. Identical twins have exactly the same genes and since only one of the twins developed the disease, then rheumatoid arthritis may not be caused by a defective gene.[11] We can conclude from this study that perhaps environmental effects, not genes, cause rheumatoid arthritis.

THE ARTHRITIS DIET

What are we to do against the toxicity of the environment, which is obviously a major aspect of the cause of arthritis? The first step in a natural health program is a good organic diet. But, the Arthritis Foundation openly warns against diets that restrict the intake of several types of foods. However, that is exactly where you have to begin with the natural treatment of all types of arthritis. Non-foods such as sugar, artificial sweeteners, food dyes, colorings, and additives must be eliminated from the diet. Sugar can be safely replaced with natural Stevia sweeteners. Refined sugar has hundreds of detrimental effects including an overgrowth of Candida albicans which produces toxic chemicals as a result of its metabolic functions. Some of these toxic chemicals can cause joint pain and inflammation.[12] Saturated animal fat should be avoided not only because it causes hardening of the arteries but because it harbors toxic chemicals picked up from the environment. Next to be reduced or eliminated are wheat products; gluten in wheat has been implicated in arthritic disease. Dairy products should also be reduced because they promote PGE2 pro-inflammatory mediators.[13,14,15] Also many people don't have sufficient lactose enzymes to digest dairy leaving incompletely digested molecules free to cause allergy reactions that can cause or aggravate arthritic symptoms.[16,17,18,19] A study in *Lanced* showed that osteoarthritis patients receiving NSAIDs exhibited greater intestinal permeability to food antigens.[20]

In a small trial of six rheumatoid arthritis patients, two of whom were obese, a low calorie, fat-free weight control formula or diet was introduced. The two obese patients remained symptom-free for 9-14 months and the other four patients also experienced a remission in symptoms. Within 24-72 hours of reintroducing vegetable oil, animal fat, cheese, safflower oil, beef, coconut oil or other foods with a high proportion of calories from fat, they experienced exacerbation of symptoms with joint swelling, morning stiffness, and tenderness.[13,14]

Foods that make a difference in arthritis are black mission figs, raw goat's milk, black cherries, green kale, celery, parsley, and apples—preferably all organic.[21] Garlic, and many other herbs, have a long history of health benefits, which include antioxidant effects on the symptoms of aging.[22,23,24]

Results of a study of people living in southern Greece suggest that eating abundant amounts of olive oil and cooked vegetables may reduce the risk of developing rheumatoid arthritis. Researchers found that people who consumed the least olive oil were 2.5 times more likely to develop rheumatoid arthritis than those who consumed the most. And those who consumed the most cooked vegetables had a 75% lower risk of developing rheumatoid arthritis. The authors suggest that antioxidant substances in both foods could play a role. Olive oil is rich in vitamin E, which has a beneficial role as a free-radical quencher, as are vegetable antioxidants such as beta-carotene and vitamin C. The typical American diet is high in saturated fats from meat that are broken down to hormones that promote inflammation. The fatty acid in olive oil, on the other hand, is broken down to hormones that inhibit inflammation.[25]

Doctors should take into account that up to fifty-one percent of rheumatoid arthritis patients, as reported in a recent study, changed their diets by reducing animal fat, sugar, and red meat, and increased their consumption of fruit and vegetables. The patients expressed a concern that they could not get diets appropriate for their disease from their hospital treatment center.[26] Doctors should also note that another recent study confirmed that some form of complementary, alternative medicine is used by over 80% of rheumatoid arthritis patients with dietary and behavioral therapies being the most commonly used.[27]

Studies investigating the association of diet and rheumatoid arthritis have been going on for decades, each time showing beneficial results with no side effects. Looking through these many studies and also calculating the thousands of patients who benefit from dietary restrictions given by natural health practitioners, one can't help wonder why such an obviously successful approach to the treatment of arthritis is not promoted widely. In a very early study of twenty-six patients with rheumatoid arthritis, all taking NSAIDs, 16 were placed on a diet of fruit and vegetable juices and herbal tea for 7-10 days (1 stopped after 2 days). Ten patients served as controls. Most of the 15 experimental patients felt better by day 5-6. At the end of the diet, 10 reported reduction in pain and stiffness. Five of fifteen showed objective improvement defined as a greater than 10% decrease in the SED (sedimentation) rate with associated decrease in joint tenderness, while only one of the controls improved.[18]

Twenty-two patients followed diets that excluded common food allergens. Twenty patients subjectively improved, and 19 reported that certain foods would repeatedly exacerbate arthritic symptoms. It took an average of ten days after food elimination for improvement to occur. When foods were reintroduced, reactions to allergic foods with worsening of symptoms varied from 2 hours to 2 weeks. The most common allergic foods were grains (14 patients); milk (4); nuts (8); beef (4); eggs (5); and 1 each for chicken, fish, potato, onion, and liver.[17] In one case study a 52 year-old white female, with an 11-year history of joint pain, tenderness, swelling and stiffness, was diagnosed with rheumatoid arthritis and was subsequently not helped by taking NSAIDs.

She was placed on a baseline diet for 6 days, a 3-day mineral water fast and vanilla flavored Vivonex. There were no notable responses to 52 placebo challenges, but she responded with symptomatic deterioration and worsening of SED rate and other peak responses to cows milk challenge on 4 separate occasions. While there was no elevation of IgE antibodies to foods, there was a mild elevation of IgG and large amounts of IgG4 anti-milk antibodies.[16]

Twenty patients were placed on a vegan diet following a 7-10 day fast. Also excluded or used sparingly were refined sugar, corn flour, salt, strong spices, alcohol, tea, and coffee. After 4 months, 12 patients reported some improvement, 5 reported no change, and 3 felt worse. Most of the improved patients felt less pain and were better able to function, although there were no changes in objective measures such as grip strength and joint tenderness.[15] In a fasting and vegetarian diet-treatment study 27 rheumatoid arthritis patients were first put on a 7-10 day partial fast which allowed vegetable broth, various spices and teas, and juices made from potato, parsley, beets, carrots, beets and celery. They were compared to a control group of 26 patients who ate an unrestricted diet. After the partial fast the treatment group introduced one food every 2 days. If the food provoked symptoms, it was removed from the diet and then reintroduced in 7 days. If the food provoked symptoms a second time, it was no longer allowed in the diet. As additional insurance against eating allergenic foods, during the first 3½ months, gluten, meat, fish, eggs, dairy products, refined sugar, citrus fruit, preservatives, coffee, tea, alcohol, salt, and strong spices were avoided. Both dairy and gluten were returned to the diet after 3½ months if they did not provoke symptoms. After 4 weeks the treatment group showed a significant improvement in the number of tender joints. Measurements were made using an articular index, number of swollen joints, pain scores, duration of morning stiffness, grip strength, SED rate, C-reactive protein, WBC count, and a health assessment questionnaire. In the control group only the pain scores improved with any significance whereas in the treatment group all measures improved.[28] The improvements were still noted in the treatment group one year later.[29]

In a study of a raw food diet, forty patients with rheumatoid arthritis were randomly assigned to receive an uncooked vegan diet or a control diet for 3 months. After this period patients on the vegan diets reported relief of stiffness, joint swelling and general well being. When the vegan group switched back to their normal omnivorous diet, most of the symptoms became worse.[30] Forty-six adults with rheumatoid arthritis were placed on a raw food diet avoiding grains and dairy products. The duration of the study was between 1-3 years. Thirty-six patients had significant improvement in painful joints, swollen joints, morning stiffness, SED rate and other parameters. Among those who had positive benefits, 17 were clearly improved and 19 were in complete remission for 1-5 years. Eight of these 19 patients stopped all medications and no relapse was noted. Seven of the people that had positive results had all of their symptoms return when they abandoned their diet, but again improved when they resumed their diet.[19]

Many researchers are writing about the need for studies on arthritis and antioxidants urging funding for this important work. One group writes about the importance of nutrition in protecting the living organism against the potentially lethal effects of reactive oxygen species and toxic environmental chemicals. The authors say that "Emerging newer concepts focus on the role of trace elements and other dietary components in antioxidant defense and detoxification mechanisms." And add that "Trace elements like iron, zinc magnesium, selenium, copper, and manganese are some of the elements involved in antioxidant defense mechanisms. Inadequate intake of these nutrients has been associated with . . . arthritis . . . where a pathogenic role of free radicals is suggested." Cautioning that "The importance of diet in the prevention of chemical-induced toxicity can not be undetermined," they emphasize that "Recent reports on the role of bioflavonoids as antioxidants and their potential use to reduce the risks of chronic disease in human beings have opened a new arena for future research."[31,32] Another group at the National Public Health Institute in Helsinki, Finland studied the association between flavonoid intake and risk of several chronic diseases, and found that the risk of some chronic diseases such as arthritis may be lower at higher dietary flavonoid intakes.[33]

ESSENTIAL FATTY ACIDS IN ARTHRITIS

Yes, trace elements, iron, zinc-magnesium, selenium, copper, and manganese; vitamins B, C, E and bioflavins; and essential fatty acids all take part in the metabolic processes of the body. They are natural and necessary cofactors in processes that keep the body healthy. Auto-immune dysfunction begins with deficiencies of these necessary nutrients and with toxins taken in from the environment.

Polyunsaturated fatty acids (PUFA) in the form of supplements have been studied for many years in the treatment of arthritis. In a 1985 study 17 patients were placed on a high PUFA, low saturated fat diet and also supplemented with 10 caps of Max EPA/day. A control group of twenty people received a typical American diet and capsules of placebo. After 12 weeks, the EPA group had significantly less morning stiffness compared to worsening symptoms in the control group. Joints were also less tender and hemoglobin improved. A rapid deterioration with increased pain and stiffness was seen in treated patients compared to controls upon cessation of the experimental diet.[34] Gil in the Faculty of Pharmacy at the University of Granada, Spain reviewed the role of polyunsaturated fatty acids (PUFA) in inflammatory disease. Acknowledging that dietary supplements of PUFA between one to eight grams per day have been beneficial in the treatment of irritable bowel disease, he also reports on recent studies in rats who have been given experimental ulcerative colitis, induced by certain chemicals, showing treatment with PUFA was able to reduce mucosal damage and inflammation.[35]

Ninety patients with rheumatoid arthritis received either 2.6 gms-omega 3 oil (fish) or placebo in a double-blind study for 12 months. The fish oil group derived significant clinical benefit on both subjective and objective pain scores.[36]

Ten patients with autoimmune disease received 300 mg of an essential oil combination EPA/DHA for periods of 3 months to 3 years. All patients were measured for levels of GLA, EPA and DHA and were found to be low. After treatment, biochemical changes showed increases in the deficiencies and marked improvement of all of their symptoms. All medications were discontinued and patients remained free of symptoms for periods up to 3 years.[37]

Another half dozen studies using fish oils showed beneficial results in the treatment of rheumatoid arthritis.[38,39,40,41,42,43] A study on fish oils found that patients were able to decrease and even discontinue their NSAIDs without experiencing a disease flare.[44]

Polyunsaturated fatty acids when taken in a dosage range of

between one to eight grams per day have been beneficial in the treatment of rheumatoid arthritis according to several studies.[45,46] A group in Australia felt fish oils should be used in such a way to prevent rheumatoid arthritis.[46] Sixty-eight percent of 43 patients described good or very good effects from simply taking one gram of cod liver oil taken for three months.[47]

A review article on rheumatoid arthritis and fish oil revealed significant benefit, including less need for anti-inflammatory drugs and decreased disease activity.[48] And studies are underway to understand the mechanism of action of Vitamin E, plant oils, and fish oils on inflammatory disease.[49]

In 1983 one of the first studies on gamma-linolenic acid (GLA) was done. GLA is found in evening primrose oil and borage oil. In this study of 20 patients with arthritis, evening primrose oil, when combined with cofactors zinc, vitamin C, B3, and B6, was as effective as conventional treatment with NSAIDs.[50] In 1989 Dr. David Horrobin found similar beneficial effects of evening primrose oil alone in the treatment of rheumatoid arthritis.[51] And Horrobin felt that treatment with gamma-linolenic acid could play an important role in all rheumatological diseases.[52]

Thirty-seven patients with rheumatoid arthritis received either 1.4 gms q.d. of GLA from borage oil or placebo (cottonseed oil). This was a double-blind trial that lasted 24 weeks. The GLA-treated group had significant reduction in signs and symptoms of disease activity whereas patients receiving the placebo showed no change in symptoms. GLA reduced the number of tender joints by 36% and tender joint score by 45%. All patients were allowed to continue with their NSAIDs during the study.[53] A review article in 1995 confirmed that gamma-linolenic acid was a useful treatment for rheumatoid arthritis.[54] Then in 1996 a study of evening primrose oil patients taking GLA over a one-year period showed progressive improvement. Sixteen of 21 patients showed statistically significant and meaningful improvement at 12 months compared with study entry.[55] Later studies in 2000 continued to show beneficial results.[56] And in 2001 we find research indicating the exact mechanism of action of these essential oils as they suppress tumor necrosis factors.[57] You may recall our discussion in Chapter Three of infliximab, an immune-suppressing drug from a class of drugs called anti-TNF (Tumor Necrosis Factor) used to treat rheumatoid arthritis and Crohn's Disease. This wildly expensive and terrifyingly toxic drug is a patented drug that does the same thing that borage oil and evening primrose oil do naturally and without side effects.

GLYCOSAMINOGLYCANS IN ARTHRITIS

Perna canaliculus (green-lipped mussel) is a rich source of glycosaminoglycans, beneficial in the treatment of rheumatoid arthritis. Twenty-eight patients with arthritis, already taking NSAIDs, were also supplemented with perna canaliculus (green-lipped mussel) 350 mg t.i.d. daily or placebo for 6 months. There was significant improvement in the experimental group as compared to controls.[58] In 1980 another study was done using 1,000 mg of perna canaliculus. This was a double blind study on 25 rheumatoid arthritis patients with an average age of 57 years. These patients had failed to respond to NSAIDs. After 3 months, 67% of treated patients versus 30% of the placebo group responded favorably. Following this the placebo-treated patients were then switched to the Perna c. and 60% of these people responded favorably.[59]

For hundreds of years many herbs have been used for the symptoms of arthritis in the form of creams, single herbs in teas or capsules and specific formulations to treat inflammation and pain. Capsicum or red pepper treats tired painful muscles and stiff joints.[60] Chimaphila umbellata improves kidney function in rheumatic patients.[61] Cimicifuga racemosa or Black cohosh treats muscular soreness and aching in osteoarthritis, and the pain of movement in the joints of the fingers and hands in rheumatoid arthritis.[62] Harpagophytum procumbens has anti-inflammatory properties.[63] It also treats pain and improves mobility.[64] It is one of the many herbs that is being currently investigated for use in arthritis. In one study, Harpagophytum not only was as effective as NSAID in the treatment of knee or hip osteoarthritis, it reduced the need for analgesic and nonsteroidal anti-inflammatory therapy and it had far less side effects.[65]

HERBAL TREATMENT OF ARTHRITIS

Smilax or Sarsaparilla has a long history of use to treat the symptoms of chronic rheumatism.[66,67] Xanthoxylum americanum or Prickly ash is used in arthritis because it stimulates circulation.[68] The herbal spice curcumin, which has been used for centuries in Ayurvedic medicine, has potent anti-inflammatory effects, especially for acute inflammation. It has been found to be equal or even more potent than cortisone and phenylbutazone in acute inflammation.[69] Ginger is a herb that increases circulation and settles the stomach. Specifically, ginger inhibits prostaglandin and leukotriene synthesis, which have an effect on inflammatory processes. It is also an antioxidant and inhibits platelet aggregation, which may explain why it seems to enhance circulation. And it contains proteases similar to bromelain which have anti-inflammatory effects.[70] In a group of 247 patients with knee osteoarthritis, a ginger extract had a statistically significant effect on reducing their symptoms. It is interesting that the only side effects with the ginger were said to be mostly mild GI reactions, whereas ginger is a well-known anti-nausea agent used for travel sickness, and nausea and vomiting of the pregnant.[71]

In a trial of 78 people with half receiving willow bark extract and half receiving placebo, researchers found that the willow bark extract showed a moderate analgesic effect in osteoarthritis and appeared to be well tolerated.[72] This study confirmed a previous one using willow bark extract on a group of patients with osteoarthritis.[73] And another group found that willow bark extract may be a useful and safe treatment for low back pain.[74]

In a study of 149 arthritis patients, 61% of patients treated with yucca extract noted less swelling, pain and stiffness as compared to 22% of a placebo group.[75] In Seoul, Korea, a group of researchers evaluated SKI 306X, a purified extract from a mixture of three oriental herbal medicines (Clematis mandshurica, Trichosanthes kirilowii and Prunella vulgaris), as a treatment for osteoarthritis and found no significant adverse events were observed in patients, and they concluded it provided clinical efficacy in the patients.[76] Another study using SKI 306X on laboratory specimens of rabbit cartilage showed that it is protective of joint cartilage tissue.[77]

HOMEOPATHIC GEL

About 180 patients with knee osteoarthritis were treated by a NSAID piroxicam gel or a homeopathic gel in a double blind study. The homeopathic gel was at least as effective and as well tolerated as the NSAID gel.[78]

GLUCOSAMINE SULFATE AND OSTEOARTHRITIS

Glucosamine sulfate, derived from the shells of shrimp and crab, has changed the face of osteoarthritis treatment over the last two decades. It is becoming the treatment of choice for those who want to avoid the use of NSAIDs and other strong medications. In 1982 there appeared one of the first studies using glucosamine for osteoarthritis. Researchers found that glucosamine sulphate was just as effective as ibuprofen, a common non-steroidal anti-inflammatory drug, in relieving the pain and inflammation of osteoarthritis. But just as important, it had little or no side effects.[79] Another group compared glucosamine sulfate to ibuprofen specifically for osteoarthritis of the knee and found the same results—that glucosamine was just as effective as ibuprofen, but without the side effects.[80] Researchers studied over 250 patients with osteoarthritis of the knee using 1,500 mg of glucosamine sulfate. They called glucosamine a slow-acting drug and concluded that it may be a safe and effective symptomatic treatment for osteoarthritis.[81] In 1994 a German research group also compared glucosamine sulfate to ibuprofen for osteoarthritis of the knee and found that glucosamine was just as effective as ibuprofen, but without the side effects.[82] When 150 patients with osteoarthritis were randomized to receive 400 mg of glucosamine sulfate or placebo intramuscularly twice weekly for 6 weeks, there was progressive improvement in symptom scores.[83]

A Chinese study compared glucosamine to ibuprofen. It confirmed that glucosamine sulfate is selective for osteoarthritis, equally as effective as non-steroidal anti-inflammatories (NSAIDs) but much better tolerated, having virtually no side effects. The authors suggest all these factors make glucosamine particularly useful in the long-term treatments needed in osteoarthritis, which is a chronic and progressive disease.[84] A

3-year, randomized, placebo-controlled, double-blind study on the use of glucosamine sulfate for knee osteoarthritis showed the long-term benefits of the supplement. There were absolutely no side effects with this treatment and the authors concluded that long-term treatment with glucosamine sulfate halted the progression of knee osteoarthritis and significantly changed the health outcomes of the group of individuals taking it.[85] In one study comparing glucosamine and the anti-inflammatory ibuprofen, both reduced pain levels in patients with TMJ degenerative joint disease. But glucosamine had a much greater influence in reducing pain produced during function and on pain caused by daily activities. Glucosamine also continued to work after treatment was stopped.[86]

Glucosamine was elevated to the status of a disease-modifying agent for osteoarthritis and not just symptom-modifying when a study showed that it prevented joint-space narrowing. In progressive osteoarthritis joint spaces narrow and are lost over time. But in a three-year period of treatment with glucosamine there was no joint-space lost compared to controls. Symptoms in the glucosamine group improved while patients on placebo had an increase in symptoms. There were also no side effects in the group on glucosamine.[87] By 2002, even though researchers were still asking the question, "Is glucosamine worth taking for osteoarthritis?," at least people in the UK were answering that question with their purses and buying glucosamine to the tune of 10 million pounds annually.[88]

CHONDROITIN SULFATE AND OSTEOARTHRITIS

Chondroitin sulfate is another safe treatment for osteoarthritis that has been actively used and studied in the past decade. In 1992 a French group studied patients with knee and hip arthritis, treating them with chondroitin sulfate for three months. Even after two months of treatment there was significant pain control. According to researchers, tolerance of chondroitin was outstanding. They declared that chondroitin sulfate is useful for the symptomatic treatment of osteoarthritis and for reducing the need for non-steroidal anti-inflammatory agents, which have far more side effects than chondroitin.[89]

In Geneva, researchers tested the effects of 800 mg daily of chondroitin sulfate on knee osteoarthritis in a 1-year, randomized, double-blind, controlled pilot study. They found it to be an effective and safe, symptomatic, slow-acting drug for the treatment of knee osteoarthritis. They also found that chondroitin seems to stabilize the joint-space width and to favorably modulate bone and joint metabolism.[90] Another group in Hungary treated osteoarthritic patients with chondroitin sulfate using 400 mg twice per day over a six-month period. The treatment had no side effects and was seen as a symptomatic slow-acting drug in knee osteoarthritis.[91] Researchers in Paris wanted to compare once-a-day dosage of 1,200 mg of chondroitin sulfate with three times a day 400 mg. They found that chondroitin improved patients' symptoms and also joint mobility. And 1,200 mg taken once a day is no different than 400 mg taken three times a day.[92]

In a journal article that reviewed six trials using glucosamine and seven using chondroitin for osteoarthritis, they are both described as effective when used alone. However, the authors suggest it is probably reasonable to use the combination for even more beneficial results.[93] A group of researchers found the combination of glucosamine and chondroitin more useful in the treatment of TMJ (tempromandibular joint syndrome) than either supplement alone.[94] The authors in one review of the literature analyzed fifteen published studies of the effects of glucosamine and chondroitin supplements on osteoarthritis. The combined results of the studies, adjusted for quality and variability in the supplements, indicated a moderate benefit from glucosamine treatment and a large benefit from chondroitin treatment.[95]

VITAMINS AND MINERALS IN ARTHRITIS TREATMENT

There are numerous and ongoing studies using various vitamins and minerals for the treatment of arthritis. They are not funded nearly to the extent that drug interventions are. And their largely positive results are never publicized to the extent that new, so-called miracle-drug breakthroughs are. Thus, we must understand how the commercialization of health and disease has led to the over-advertising of drugs. We must continue to read and study alternative health materials and determine for ourselves whether diet, supplements, herbs and other natural interventions are in fact the most commonsense approach to our health.

A study in the Annals of Rheumatology showed that a diet rich in vitamin C, E and beta carotene may slow the progression of osteoarthritis. They said that people taking "middling to high doses" of vitamin C reduced their risk for osteoarthritis by three-fold. Those taking the highest amounts of vitamin C had less risk of developing knee pain. The next vitamin that reduced the risk of osteoarthritis was beta carotene, and vitamin E proved beneficial for men. Those who took vitamin D had a reduced risk of osteoarthritis progression, but not disease prevention. The researchers suggested that these supplements should be used in addition to glucosamine sulfate and chondroitin sulfate.[96]

One group found that chronic inflammation lowers antioxidant vitamin levels in rheumatoid arthritis. They also found that the combination of low antioxidant vitamin levels and the presence of a chronic inflammatory process and low density lipoprotein may explain the high risk of cardiovascular disease in patients with rheumatoid arthritis.[97] A small group of 20 patients was studied in a double-blind trial comparing 6 mg/day boron with a placebo. The trial occurred over an eight-week period. Of the 10 patients on boron, 5 improved. Only 1 of 10 in the placebo group improved. The boron had a significant benefit for those patients with severe osteoarthritis. There were no side effects.[98]

In 1955, Dr. William Kaufman reported on 663 patients who received niacinamide (a B vitamin) in the dose range of 2-3,000 mg per day (taken along with a B-complex 100 mg) for the treatment of osteoarthritis. Compared to an untreated group of 842 patients, the osteoarthritis group showed superior scores on an index of joint range of movement.[99] In a follow-up report Kaufman wrote about niacinamide and called it a most neglected vitamin. Deficiency of another B vitamin, pantothenic acid, is associated with osteoarthritis according to early studies in rats. An acute deficiency of pantothenic acid in rats resulted in joint change pathology that mirrored osteoarthritis with calcification of cartilage and formation of osteophytes.[100] In a group of 66 rheumatoid arthritis patients, the blood levels of pantothenic acid were significantly lower than a group of controls. And the lower the level of pantothenic acid, the greater the severity of arthritis. It was further noted that normal patients who ate vegetables had a much higher pantothenate level than normals on a usual balanced diet.[101]

In another study, eighteen patients with rheumatoid arthritis were given 2 grams of calcium pantothenate daily by mouth. Another group was treated with placebo. After two months patients in the experimental group showed a significant reduction in morning stiffness. The control group did not report improvement.[102] A study using IM calcium-D-pantothenate had temporary improvement of symptoms. Royal jelly, rich in pantothenic acid, was added to their regime. After 28 days of pantothenate injections and royal jelly, 70% of the patients noted general improvement, increased joint mobility, a fall in SED rate, and increased blood levels of pantothenate. Ten vegetarians were treated with the same regime and they improved by the fourteenth day and experienced a greater rise in whole blood pantothenate levels than non-vegetarian arthritics.[101]

Vitamin C and osteoarthritis was studied in the 1980's and showed beneficial results. One review article says that it is indicated for the treatment of osteoarthritis at the cellular level.[103] An animal experimental study found that cartilage from osteoarthritic guinea pigs fed very low vitamin C daily (2-4 mg) showed classic signs of advanced osteoarthritis compared with a group of controls fed 150 mg daily. The group on the higher amount of vitamin C had much less cartilage erosion and milder cell and biochemical changes around their osteoarthritic joints.[104] Studies done in the laboratory showed that ascorbic acid had a growth effect on rabbit chondrocytes.[105] And in another study using both human and rabbit chondrocytes, additional ascorbic acid was found necessary for growth.[106] White blood cell and plasma levels of ascorbate are consistently lower in rheumatoid arthritis patients.[107] This is especially so in the case of patients consuming daily doses of aspirin.[108] Some researchers feel this is due to the increased rates of oxidation of ascorbate in the ongoing inflammation of rheumatoid arthritis.[109]

In 1978 vitamin E was found to be a prostaglandin inhibitor just like NSAIDs. Twenty-nine patients were divided into two groups. One group first received 600 mg of tocopherol and the other a placebo for ten days. 2% had a "good analgesic effect" compared to 4% on placebo.[110] A later study corroborated those results.[104] The authors of another study on vitamin E and rheumatoid arthritis found a small but significant analgesic activity, which they felt complemented standard anti-inflammatory treatment.[111]

A clinical trial of zinc was undertaken with twenty-four rheumatoid arthritis patients who were not helped by conventional treatments. Twelve patients received 50 mg zinc 3x daily for 12 weeks while the rest received placebo. There were significant improvements in joint swelling, morning stiffness, walking time and subjective symptoms during the first part of the study with continuing impressive improvement in the second part in both groups when the placebo group was also treated with zinc.[112] A double-blind crossover study on a group of 24 psoriatic arthritis patients was undertaken using 220 mg of zinc sulphate three times per day for six weeks. There was reduction of joint pain in the first six weeks and further improvement in morning stiffness and overall condition during a further 24 weeks of study.[113] In an observational study, a group of 28 patients matched with controls showed a significantly lower level of serum zinc and a higher 24-hour urinary zinc loss.[114] Case reports on the benefits of zinc therapy in arthritis appeared in Carl Pfeiffer's book *Zinc and Other Micro-Nutrients*.[115]

In a book titled *Medical Nutrition from Marz*, there is a report on an unpublished study in Poona, India. Eighteen rheumatoid arthritis patients were divided into two groups. Half were given 250 mg of zinc sulfate (50 mg of elemental zinc) three times a day. The zinc-treated group showed significant improvement in joint swelling, joint tenderness, morning stiffness, onset of fatigue, general condition of the patient, and 50-foot walking time. At cross-over, a similar response was observed in the placebo group when they were given a trial of zinc. Patients were also able to cut back their NSAID by half.[116]

A clinical trial comparing a copper supplement to aspirin showed that copper salicylate was more effective than either salicylic acid or copper acetate and produced reduction in morning stiffness, increased joint mobility, and reduced need for other drugs.[117] An earlier trial by the same group showed an 89% improvement in 1140 patients treated with short-term IV copper salicylate. They experienced remission of fever, increased joint mobility, decreased swelling and normalization of SED rate for over a time span of about three years.[118] Reviews by several authors found that copper salicylates were the best copper complex for the treatment of arthritic pain.[119,120,121,122] Animal studies showed that copper salicylate had both an anti-inflammatory and an analgesic effect on arthritic rats.[123] Even the "old wives tales" about copper bracelets helping arthritis pain may have some validity. In a crossover study of 240 arthritis patients, one group wore a copper bracelet for 1 month followed by a placebo bracelet for one month. Group two wore the placebo first and then the copper bracelet. A third group wore no bracelets. A greater number of people thought the copper bracelets gave them relief. And those who wore copper and improved began to deteriorate when they were switched to the placebo bracelets. The bracelets were weighed for copper loss and the average loss was 13 mg.[124]

Selenium is a trace mineral that is often decreased in rheumatoid arthritis. In one study of 26 girls with juvenile arthritis, selenium blood levels were lower than controls. Blood glutathione peroxidase was also slightly lower and was lowest in patients with the most severe disease.[125] In another study eighty-seven rheumatoid arthritis patients had significantly lower serum selenium levels than controls. And again levels were lowest in patients with the more active and disabling forms of the disease.[126] A study using selenium supplementation in a group of rheumatoid arthritis patients showed less tender or swollen joints, and morning stiffness. Patients needed less cortisone and NSAIDs than controls. There were also decreases in laboratory indicators of inflammation (C-reactive protein, alpha 2-globuline, prostaglandin E2). There were no side effects with treatment. The authors concluded that selenium can be considered as an additional treatment to patients with rheumatoid arthritis.[127]

Sulfur may be a deficiency in rheumatoid arthritis patients. A sulfur amino acid, cystine, measured in fingernails is normal at 12% but in rheumatoid arthritis patients the level is only 8.9%.[128] Early experimental studies on rheumatoid arthritis and IV colloidal sulphur showed disappearance of pain and effusion and return of fingernail cystine to normal.[129,130]

Twenty-five rheumatoid arthritis patients with moderate to severe symptoms were placed on small maintenance doses of steroids and also 20-40 mg of bromelain (a natural enzyme found in papaya and pineapple) 3 pills four times a day. It was found, after 13 weeks, that 28% had excellent results, 45% had good results, 14% had fair results, and 14% had poor results with this regime.[131]

UNSAPONIFIABLES IN ARTHRITIS THERAPY

Avocado/soybean unsaponifiables (sometimes called ASU) are extracted from a mixture of avocado and soybean oil (in a ratio of either one or two parts of avocado oil to three parts of soybean) The main theory is that ASU might be able to affect the development and repair of cartilage.[132] In a three-month trial of avocado/

soybean unsaponifiables the treatment group had less pain and used less NSAIDs than the placebo group. Overall patient ratings were significantly better in the ASU group and there were no side effects.[133] A prospective, randomized, double-blind, placebo-controlled, multicenter clinical trial was done on 164 patients over a six-month period using avocado/soybean unsaponifiables. Half of the group received ASU and half a placebo. Pain decreased by about one half, NSAID intake was lower, and the success rate was 39% in the ASU group and 18% in the placebo group. The authors noted that overall functional disability was significantly reduced in the ASU group. And the greatest improvement appeared in patients with hip osteoarthritis. There were no side effects with this treatment.[134] In another 3-month study using ASU all test indicators showed significant improvement. Dosage of NSAIDs and analgesics decreased by more than 50% in 71% of the patients receiving ASU compared to 36% of the patients receiving placebo.[135]

HYDROTHERAPY IN ARTHRITIS

A study to determine the effects of bathing in the Dead Sea on rheumatoid arthritis showed improvement in morning stiffness, patient self-assessment, right and left grip, Schober test, and distance from finger to floor when bending forward. Other symptoms such as tender and swollen joints, and inflammatory neck and back pain, improved over time and were much better in a subgroup that also had mud packs and sulfur baths in addition to sun, ultraviolet exposure and Dead Sea baths.[136] This study emphasizes the need for hydrotherapy in the treatment of arthritis. Such treatments can include Epsom salts baths, mud packs, sea clay wraps, and massage.

LEECHES WORK FOR OSTEOARTHRITIS

Treating osteoarthritis with leeches may seem medieval but a 2001 study in the *Annals of Rheumatic Diseases* showed that the tiny blood-sucking creatures can help relieve chronic pain caused by osteoarthritis. Ten people with osteoarthritis had pain relief and no side effects. Pain was significantly reduced for up to 4 weeks. The leeches were left on the patients' knees for 80 minutes. And the leeches produced faster pain relief than conventional drugs given to patients in a control group. Not only were the treatments removing blood but they were giving back saliva, which contains analgesic and anaesthetic compounds, as well as hirudin, an anti-blood clotting agent.[137]

CONCLUSION

We know that scientific research only measures one variable at a time. That's why diet studies in the treatment of arthritis are so important: When one nutrient is measured and shown to be only slightly effective that nutrient is tossed aside. So trying to fit nutrients into the scientific-testing box only serves to minimize their importance. Often nutrient studies last only a few weeks whereas a patient might have had a nutrient deficiency for many years. Also, the body works in synergy and requires all the nutrients to be working in concert. Giving only one nutrient at a time is not a valid test of the body's function and researchers don't seem to recognize that simple, commonsense fact.

We have presented many studies on the use of nutrients in arthritis ranging over the past seventy years and they each come to the same conclusion. They confirm that diet, essential fatty acids, certain minerals, and vitamins are all beneficial for the treatment of arthritis. Each and every study says that the nutrient being studied can and should be used as an additional treatment for arthritis. Yet, each study also says that further research is necessary, making the reader think that no conclusion has been drawn. But don't be confused, that statement is probably made to make sure their research funding continues. But we think it is safe to say, looking at seventy years of research, that the millions of dollars spent on continuing this research is ill-spent; instead it should be used to make supplements available to everyone with arthritis, and everyone with chronic disease. That move alone will save the country billions of dollars in health care costs and loss of work. It will also save the dignity and the health of millions.

5

PROTOCOL FOR ARTHRITIS

Now that we've discussed the causes of arthritis and its alternative therapies, it's time to lay out a definitive protocol for helping the arthritic condition. It is important to note that the suggested activities, nutrients, foods, and herbs should be taken incrementally. In other words, one should begin taking these suggested items either in smaller doses at first, increasing the dosages each week, or by taking a few (2-3) items initially, increasing the amount of items taken overall.

Any person beginning this protocol should first be diagnosed by a licensed physician for the condition that we are discussing. Treatment and medications must be considered in determining if any of the suggested vitamins, minerals, foods, and herbs are contraindicated. Special considerations should be given to pregnant and nursing mothers.

DETOXIFICATION

The very first step that should take place in this protocol is detoxification. If one has not been a vegetarian or even has a habit of eating out at restaurants frequently, chances are the colon needs to be conditioned and cleansed properly in order to maximize nutrient absorption. Restaurant food can be a source of parasite infection. Colon cleansing is an ancient technique that dates back as far as the Egyptians. Hippocrates was a teacher of colon conditioning, which helps heal and restore the colon to its proper shape and function.

A great formula for colon conditioning is a drink made from ground flax seeds, psyllium seeds, and a liquid clay called liquid bentonite. This special clay helps absorb toxins. Use one table-spoon of each of the seeds combined with one (1)cup bentonite. Stir quickly and drink before it gels. This mixture should be taken two hours before eating meals, every four hours throughout the day for three day. Do not exceed three days twice a month.

Otherwise, seek out a good colon hydrotherapist in your area. Begin a program of conditioning the colon. This will help the absorption of nutrients in order to kick-start the program.

CLEANSING AT HOME

Drink lots of water
Make sure the water you're drinking is either filtered, distilled ionized or passed through a reverse osmosis system, (a type of fil-tration). As with the nutrients, one should slowly increase the intake of water as well, eventually consuming one gallon per day.

Take a hot bath
Saunas are popular throughout the world for their detoxification effects, especially in Norwegian countries. But did you know that taking hot baths could be just as effective at releasing toxins from the body? If you are not conditioned enough to perspire during your aerobic work-outs, which means you either can not put enough intensity into the work out or your endurance is not yet enough to maintain movement for an extended period of time,

then you can still help your body cleanse by taking hot baths. Start by soaping yourself clean with a pre-cleanse in either a shower or regular bath. Once you're skin is clean, fill the tub with water, as hot as you could possibly bear without scolding yourself. Begin with a five-minute bath where you are completely immersed in the water throughout the entire hot-bath session. Some people don't realize the effectiveness of such a detoxification and upon completing the initial bath feel a little sick from releasing too many toxins. Once again, as with all the other parts of this protocol, begin slowly and build through time. Don't expect miracles to happen by pushing yourself and doing too much at once. This can only hurt you. Build yourself up to a thirty-minute regimen, by adding five-minutes to each session, three to four times per week.

Some herbs that you might consider adding to the baths are: catnip, peppermint, blessed thistle, and horsetail. Prepare one cup of tea from the herbs per bath. If you find that you are sensitive to the herbs or have too quick a detox from the herbs, just take hot-baths with plain water.

It is advisable to consume about 1000-mg. of vitamin C and one 8-oz. glass of fresh room temperature water during the hot-bath sessions.

Exercise

The second element of the protocol is exercise. Where it is recommended to exercise 5-6 days a week for 60 minutes aerobically, we must assume that the individual beginning the program is not fit enough to exercise for such an extended period initially, and so exercise must begin with 10 minutes and increase gradually by 10-15% per week. The same holds true for supplements. One must increase 10-15% from the amount taken in the beginning, steadily maintaining the program with the aim of doing the full program in due time. Do not rush this program; rather, make it a lifestyle, incorporating stress management techniques and self-empowerment philosophies. I have an entire library of over 100 self-empowerment videos and audiocassettes. Some of these titles can be previewed on www.garynull.com.

Consider that your heart pumps blood throughout your body allowing nutrients to travel to vital cells along with oxygen. That same blood then takes waste materials from the cells to the lungs, liver and kidneys. Other toxic matter is then filtered or exhaled through the lungs in the form of carbon dioxide. But what about the lymphatic system? The lymphatic system aids in the cleansing process, which results in a healthier immune function. This is directly related to the arthritic condition. The problem is that there is no pump for the lymphatic system. The only way to successfully circulate lymph fluid, which carries much of the toxic waste matter from the cells, is through bodily movements such as walking, trampolining, running, or any other form of exercise that has a "bounce" to it. Unfortunately, people with arthritis, in many cases, have troubles with their knees making "high impact" or even "low impact" exercises almost impossible. No worries. Yoga and vigorous, lightweight training are beneficial as well. Water aerobics is a great alternative to ground aerobics. The main idea in creating a regimen to help lymphatic circulation is to flex muscles in ways that cause a pumping action throughout the body. Build up to 1-hour per day of aerobic exercise. Take your pulse throughout your aerobic work-out to make sure you are neither under nor over exerting yourself. Generally, your target rate is determined by taking 220 and subtracting your age and then multiplying the result by 70 percent. So a 31 year old person would have a rate of 220 minus 31 times 70 percent or 132.

In addition to aerobic exercise you must do weight training 3 times per week. There are plenty of exercise videos on the market that present fitness routines that use light-weights and almost non-impacting movements. Some exercises to keep high on your list of choices are: Pilates, Power Yoga, walking and weight training. These are all beneficial for the arthritic condition. Buy a book on weight lifting or better yet consult a professional trainer for some exercise tips; just get your body moving with the intention of increasing muscular intensity. This will eventually help strengthen cardiovascular strength and endurance as well as move lymph fluid for cleansing. Begin with 10 minutes of exercise per day, 5-6 days per week, eventually increasing to one-hour per day.

BEGIN THE ELIMINATION DIET

You may select from the foods listed below. Begin by eliminating, one by one: all dairy, meat, chicken, wheat, sugar, all bleached foods such as white flour, and all hydrogenated oils. I suggest that you cook at home using filtered water. Good oils such as macadamia oil, olive oil, coconut oil and safflower or sesame oil should be used in cooking. Never fry foods (but you may sauté). Steaming is the best way to prepare all vegetables. Please remember not to over-steam. Vegetables taste better al dente, and they retain more of their nutrients that way. Listed below are foods that are exceptionally beneficial for the arthritic condition. This program is not about dieting per se. There is no limit to the food that should be consumed but bear in mind that over-consumption of even a good thing will lead to excessive weight gain.

When eating, try to masticate your food thoroughly. Eat slowly and mindfully. Paying conscious attention leads to greater enjoyment of the meal. If you feel like helping yourself to a second serving of food, wait twenty minutes and then see if you're still hungry. You might be surprised to notice that you feel satisfied after twenty minutes even though you felt like helping yourself to a second portion earlier.

Begin the program by implementing the detox protocol outlined below. Go slowly! When you are ready, feel free to incorporate suggestions from the arthritis protocol listed after the detox protocol as well.

DETOX PROTOCOL

The First Four Weeks:
Two (2)—(10 oz.) glasses of green juice per day:
Juice 4 oz. dark & light green vegetables. Add 6 oz. water

Or

1 tablespoon of powdered dry green concentrate. Add 10 oz
    water
In the above juices, add 1 oz. of aloe concentrate and add one
    teaspoon of red fruit (dried concentrate).

At night:
Antioxidant complex Follow the instructions on the label
Garlic with cayenne powder Follow the instructions on the
    label
Psyllium bifidis fiber Follow the instructions on the label
Vitamin C 2500—5000 mg

After 4 weeks add:
Quercetin 550 mg three times a day
Pycnogenol 50 mg three times per day
L-Carnitine 250 mg twice a day

After 4 more weeks add:

Brain complex, 3 capsules per day or

Ginkgo Biloba 100 mg (Consult your doctor if on blood thinners)

L-Phenylalanine 75 mg

L-Glutathione 25 mg

L-Taurine 50 mg

Choline Bitartrate Complex 75 mg

Inositol 25 mg

L-Glutamine 25 mg

L-Tyrosine 25 mg

Phosphatidyl Serine 25 mg

Naturleaf (enzyme enhanced)

Plant-Sprout sterols/sitosterolins 500 mg. 4 × daily

MGN 3 500 mg. 3 × daily

Increase antioxidant complex to 5 times per day

B Complex 50 mg

DIETARY GUIDELINES

1. **No meat, including: beef, poultry, and shellfish.**
   - *Replace with*: cold water fish (tuna, salmon, trout, mackerel, sardines, cod) 4 times/week; nuts, nut butters, seeds, soybeans and soy products, organic eggs, Quinoa (high protein grain): mix grains with beans.

2. **No Dairy, including milk, yogurt, cheese, butter, ice cream, and cream sauces.**
   - *Replace with*: rice milk, soy milk, almond milk, Amazake, Silken tofu, oat milk. Nothing with "casein" in the ingredients.

3. No caffeine or alcohol, including. chocolate, coffee, tea, wines, hard liquoeur, etc.
   - *Replace with:* herb teas, grain beverages (postum, cafix, Rajas's cup), lemon water, green tea.

4. No sugar/artificial sweeteners.
   - *Replace with:* stevia root, raw honey, molasses, brown rice syrup, beet sugar and natural fruit sweetners. May use chromium Picolinate (200 mcg.) for sugar cravings.

5. No carbonated drinks, including sodas and, seltzer.
   - *Replace with:* spring water, distilled water, filtered water or fresh squeezed organic fruit juice.

6. No bread or wheat.
   - *Replace with:* spelt bread, sprouted whole grain bread, rice bread, Essene bread. Read the labels.

7. No non-organic produce.
   - *Replace with:* organic produce, include potatoes (NOT Idaho), squash, sweet potatoes, yams, grains, beans, fruits, vegetables.

8. No fried or processed foods.
   - *Replace with:* Steamed, sautéed, stir fried, grilled, broiled meals. Oils for cooking: coconut, macadamia, safflower oils. For baking: hazelnut, macadamia nut. For salads: Walnut, flax seed. Extra virgin cold pressed olive oil is okay to add to cooked foods; avoid cooking with the olive oil.

9. No food additives, preservatives, coloring agents, flavorings, MSG, or miso.

REMEMBER:
Eat primarily during the day. Have your large meal between 1 pm and 3 pm. Have a very light breakfast and a light dinner, which might include grains and any salad with dressing, sea vegetable, and/or soup.

ORGANIC MEAL PROGRAM
Quality protein and amino acids $9/10$ gram per kilogram of body weight per day, approximately 60 grams per day for women and 80 gm per day for malesmen.

SUGGESTION:
Begin by getting your protein from grains, legumes, and seeds. If needed, protein powder supplements are useful in guaranteeing sufficient amounts. The diet should provide you with 40-50 grams of fiber per day.

Choose from the following:
- Tofu &Tempeh
- Grains & Sprouts: Millet, Buckwheat, Brown Rice, Spelt, Rye, Quinoa
- Organic raw vegetables and fruits—all types
- Fatty Deep Water Fish: Cod, Tuna, Sole, Salmon or Sardines 6-8 oz.
- Raw Seeds, Raw Nuts
- Tubers: Yams, Potatoes, or Sweet Potatoes
- 3-4 servings of the Cruciferous vegetables daily: Broccoli, Cabbage, Cauliflower & Onions
- Sea Vegetables

Drink a minimum of 1 gallon of liquids, which include purified water and juice.

1-2 cups green tea daily.
Lemon juices daily—to alkalize the body.
Digestive enzymes for fatigue.

If candida is present—use grapefruit seed extract 5-10 drops in water 3X/day

ADDITIONAL DIETARY CONSIDERATIONS AND HERBS

You may choose from the following:
- Cantaloupe
- English Walnut
- Avocado
- Camu Camu
- Cucumber
- Safflower
- Black cumin
- Apricot
- Sunflower
- Butternut
- Calabash gourd
- Brazilnut
- Sesame
- Pinyon pine
- Chilgoza pine
- Olive Oil 2 tbs/day
- Cat's Claw 100 mg
- Ginger 100 mg
- Buchu Leaf 25 mg
- Horse Tail 25 mg
- Yucca 25 mg
- Tumeric 200 mg

- Sea Cucumber 300 mg
- Green Lipped Mussel 100 mg
- Garlic 2,000 mg
- Cayenne 15 mg
- Naturleaf (enzyme enhanced)
- Plant-Sprout sterols/sitosterolins 500 mg 4X/day

BENEFICIAL SUPPLEMENTATION FOR ARTHRITIS

Take the following daily in divided doses:
- Glucosamine Sulfate 1,000 mg
- Chondroitin Sulfate 500 mg
- Silica 50 mg
- Manganese 25 mg
- L-Cysteine 500 mg
- L-Glutamic Acid 200 mg
- L-Taurine 200 mg
- Boron 5 mg
- B-Complex 100 mg
- Vitamin E 400 IU
- Calcium Citrate 1,200 mg
- Magnesium Citrate 1,200 mg
- Co-Q-10 200 mg
- DMG 150 mg
- TMG 150 mg
- SOD 500 mg
- Beta Carotene 50,000 IU
- Folic Acid 1,000 mcg
- DPLA 250 mg
- Zinc 50 mg
- Digestive Enzymes As directed

- MGN 3 1500 mg
- Omega-3 3 teaspoons
- Evening Primrose Oil 2,000 mg
- Vitamin C 5,000-20,000/day
- MSM 3,000 mg/day
- GLA 920 mg/day
- DHA 1000 mg/day

TO REDUCE INFLAMMATION, TAKE:

- Perilla Oil 1,000 mg/day
- N-acetyl-D-glucosamine 500 mg/day
- Boswella acids 300 mg/day
- Shark Cartilage 750 mg/day
- Serrapeptase enzyme 5 mg/day

6

RECIPES

Blueberry Oatmeal with Soy Yogurt

½ cup oats
1 cup purified water
¼ cup fresh or frozen blueberries
¼ cup plain soy yogurt
1 Tbsp maple syrup (optional)

1. In a small sauce pan bring oats, water and blueberries to simmer and lower heat. Cook for about five to seven minutes, until oats and creamy and cooked.
2. Immediately before serving, stir in yogurt and maple syrup.

Puffed Grain Breakfast

⅓ cup puffed millet
⅓ cup puffed brown rice
⅓ cup puffed corn
2 Tbsp raw sliced almonds
1 tsp raw sunflower seeds
1 cup plain soy yogurt
½ tsp bee pollen (optional)

1. Mix the first six ingredients together. Top with bee pollen and serve.

Quinoa Pancakes

¾ cup quinoa flour
¼ cup rolled oats
½ tsp baking soda
1 tsp baking powder
1 each egg replacer
½ cup fresh extracted apple juice
½ cup soymilk
2 Tbsp safflower oil

1. Mix together quinoa flour, oats, baking soda, baking powder and egg replacer. Add juice, soymilk and oil.
2. Pour ¼ cup of batter onto a medium heat non-stick skillet. Turn the cake as they rise and bubble. Cook for an additional minute. Serve with maple syrup or warm molasses.

Seven Grain Cereal with Peaches

2½ cups water
1 cup multigrain cereal
1 each peach, pitted and one inch diced
¼ tsp cinnamon
2 Tbsp brown rice syrup

1. Bring water to a boil and slowly whisk in cereal. Let simmer for 15 minutes, stirring occasionally.
2. Add peaches, cinnamon and rice syrup. Serve immediately.

II. SMOOTHIES AND JUICES

All Green

½ each cucumber
1 leaf kale
½ bunch parsley
1 small romaine
3 stalks celery
2 ounces whole aloe vera juice

1. Juice cucumber, kale, parsley, romaine, and celery, than add aloe juice.

Chef Notes:
Buy whole leaf aloe vera juice.
To preserve juice for 24 hours, add ⅛ tsp ascorbic acid.

Apple, Carrot, and Ginger Juice

½ inch fresh ginger
3 each apples
1 each carrot

1. Juice ginger, apples, and carrots.

Chef Notes:
You may add more ginger or cut back.

Banana, Peanut Butter, and Carob Smoothie

12 ounces plain soymilk
1 each banana, peeled
2 Tbsp natural peanut butter
1 Tbsp flax oil
2 Tbsp roasted carob powder
1 Tbsp almond sliced soaked overnight in water
1 scoop protein powder

1. Blend soymilk, banana, peanut butter, and oil until smooth. Add almonds and protein powder. Drink.

Chocolate Coconut Smoothie

1 1/2 cups rice milk
1 each banana
1 Tbsp coconut oil
2 Tbsp cocoa powder
1 scoop plain or vanilla protein powder
2 tsp unsweetened shredded coconut

1. Blend rice milk with banana, oil, cocoa powder, and protein powder. Garnish with shredded coconut.

Mango Strawberry Smoothie

1 1/2 cups mango juice
1 pint strawberries
1 scoop protein powder
1/2 cup plain soy yogurt

1. Blend all ingredients until smooth.

Peach and Honey Smoothie

1 cup sliced frozen peaches
12 ounces soymilk
1 Tbsp raw honey
1 scoop protein powder

1. Blend all ingredients until smooth.

Watermelon Lemon Juice

12 1½ cups fresh extracted watermelon juice
½ lemon juiced

1. Mix both juices and drink.

Chef Notes:
Do not remove seeds from watermelon or lemons. Put them through the juicer with the fruits. This is a great juice after a long workout.

III. SOUPS

Adzuki Bean Soup

1 cup Adzuki beans, sorted and washed
6 cups vegetarian beef base
¼ cup onions, ½ inch diced
¼ cup carrots, ½ inch diced
1 each bay leaf

1. Simmer beans covered in stock with onions, carrots, and bay leaf for 1½. Occasionally skim any foam that will rise on the surface.
2. Allow beans to cool halfway and pulse in a blender until desired consistency. If soup is to thick add some water or stock to thin.

Easy Mushroom Miso Soup

1/2 cup shitake mushrooms, de-stemmed, and sliced
1/2 lb firm tofu, 1/2 inch diced
1 piece kelp, broken into 1 inch pieces
2 cups vegetable stock/soup
1 Tbsp barley miso
3 each green onions, sliced

1. Place mushrooms, tofu, and kelp into stock and simmer for five minutes.
2. Remove from heat and add miso and onions and serve.

Potato Mustard Soup

3 cups vegetable stock/soup
1 lb Yukon Gold potatoes, quartered
1/2 cup onions, 1 inch diced
1 sprig thyme
1 cup rice milk
3 Tbsp grained Dijon mustard

1. Place vegetable stock in a pot with potatoes, onions, and thyme. Bring to a simmer and cook covered for 30 minutes or until potatoes are cooked.
2. Add rice milk and mustard then puree until smooth, serve.

Quinoa Vegetable Soup

¼ cup quinoa, white or black
½ cup water
2 cups vegetable stock/soup
¼ cup carrots, ¼ inch diced
¼ cup onions, ¼ inch diced
2 tsp garlic, chopped
1 each bay leaf
1 tsp parsley, chopped
½ tsp thyme, chopped

1. Begin by washing quinoa. Bring water to boil and add quinoa. Lower to a simmer and cook quinoa slowly for about 10 minutes; do not stir. Quinoa is finished when it is tender, do not over cook or it will become a mush consistency.
2. In a soup pot, bring stock to a simmer, add remaining ingredients and simmer for 10 minutes.
3. Before serving add quinoa.

IV. SALADS

Apple, Walnut, and Tofu Salad

¼ cup onions, minced
¼ cup celery, minced
2 tsp raw apple cider vinegar
½ cup Nayonaise
¼ tsp ground, cumin
1 each apple, ½ inch diced
1 lb firm tofu, drained and crumbled
¼ cup raw walnuts

1. Combine onions, celery, vinegar, Nayonaise, cumin and apple and mix well.
2. Mix in tofu and walnuts. Serve or refrigerate for up to three days.

Beet Salad

1 tsp raw unfiltered apple cider vinegar
2 Tbsp sunflower oil
1 tsp flax oil
1 Tbsp tofu mayonnaise
¼ cup onion, diced ¼ inch
1 each apple, cored and diced ½ inch
2 cups beets, shredded
¼ cup walnuts pieces, toasted

1. In a bowl mix vinegar, oils, and tofu mayonnaise. Add onion, apple and beets.
2. Serve and top with walnuts.

Caesar Salad

1 medium head romaine lettuce
½ pint cherry tomatoes
1 recipe Caesar Dressing

1. Cut Romaine head perpendicular in one inch pieces. Wash very well in a bowl of water and spin dry.
2. Toss and with cherry tomatoes and Caesar Dressing. Serve.

Caesar Dressing

1½ cups Nayonaise, or other soy mayonnaise substitute
1 Tbsp lemon juice
2 tsp red wine vinegar
1 tsp Dijon Mustard
1 tsp capers
1 tsp anchovy filets, chopped
1 Tbsp vegan parmesan cheese
1 tsp coarse black pepper, freshly ground
pinch cayenne pepper

1. Combine all ingredients and mix well. Serve or refrigerate for up to five days.

Mixed Sprouts with Carrot Ginger Dressing

Assorted sprouts such as:
Bean, sunflower, chickpea, radish, buckwheat etc.
Optional: romaine lettuce, washed and chopped
1 recipe Carrot Ginger Dressing

1. Toss sprouts and or romaine with carrot ginger dressing.

Carrot Ginger Dressing

2 cups carrots, sliced and cooked
1/2 cup ginger, sliced
1/4 cup onions, diced
1/2 cup rice vinegar
1/4 cup Braggs Liquid Aminos
1/4 cup purified water
1/2 cup sunflower oil

1. In a food processor puree all ingredients. Chill and serve.

Carrot Raisin Salad

1/2 cup raisins, soaked overnight in water
2 cups carrots, shredded
1/4 cup Nayonaise
1/4 cup Basic Vinaigrette

1. Drain the raisins and mix with carrots, Nayonaise and
   Basic Vinaigrette.
2. Serve or refrigerate for later use.

Red Onion and Cucumber Salad

1 tsp garlic, chopped
1 tsp thyme, chopped
2 tsp rice wine vinegar
2 Tbsp sunflower oil
1 medium red onion, halved and ¼ inch sliced
2 medium cucumbers, split and ½ inch sliced
to taste black pepper

1. In as bowl mix garlic, thyme, vinegar, and oil. Toss in onion and cucumbers. Let salad marinate in refrigerator for at least eight hours.
2. With a pepper mill twist some black pepper to taste and serve.

V. BASIC DRESSINGS AND SAUCES

Basic Vinaigrette

1 tbsp tahinni
1 tbsp Dijon Mustard
1 tbsp raw honey
¼ cup raw unfiltered apple cider vinegar
¾ cup sunflower oil

1. Blend tahinni, mustard, and honey until mixed, about 10 seconds. Slowly drizzle in oil while blender is on low.

Curry Vinaigrette

1 tbsp tahinni
1 tbsp Dijon Mustard
2 tsp Madras Curry powder
1/4 cup raw unfiltered apple cider vinegar
1 Tbsp shallots, chopped
1 tsp mint, chopped
1/8 tsp ground cumin
3/4 cup sunflower oil

1. In a bowl mix tahinni, mustard, curry, vinegar, shallots, mint and cumin. While whisking slowly drizzle in oil. This dressing can be stored for up to five days.

Honey Mustard Vinaigrette and Mayonnaise

1/3 cup raw honey
1/3 cup Dijon Mustard
1/3 cup unfiltered raw apple cider vinegar
1 1/2 cups sunflower oil

1. In a blender, blend honey, mustard and vinegar for 15 seconds.
2. Drizzle in oil while blender is on low. If the mixture gets to thick to blend add two tablespoons of water at a time and continue.

For vinaigrette add 1/3 cup water to thin consistency.

Miso Tamari Vinaigrette

1 Tbsp white miso
1/4 cup rice vinegar
2 Tbsp tamari
1/2 tsp chopped garlic
1 tsp chopped cilantro and or mint
1/4 tsp sesame seeds
3/4 cup light sesame or safflower oil

1. Place all ingredients in a bowl and whisk.

Tartar Sauce

1/2 cup Nayonaise
1 Tbsp nitrate free pickles, minced
1 Tbsp capers
1 tsp lemon juice
1/2 tsp tarragon, chopped
1/2 tsp chives, chopped
1 tsp parsley, chopped
pinch cayenne pepper

1. Combine all ingredients and mix well. Serve or refrigerate for up to 4 days.

VI. VEGETABLES

Asparagus w/ Curry Vinaigrette

1 lb asparagus
1 recipe curry vinaigrette

1. Wash and cut asparagus to fit into a pot.
2. Bring a pot of water to a boil and cook asparagus for one minute.
3. Toss asparagus with vinaigrette and serve hot or cold.

Broccoli w/ Honey Dijon

2 cups broccoli florets, washed
1 recipe Honey Dijon Dressing

1. Steam broccoli lightly and cool.
2. Toss with Honey Dijon and serve or refrigerate for later

Chipolte Polenta

2 cups vegetable stock
1/2 cup corn polenta
3 Tbsp sunflower oil
1/4 cup vegan parmesan cheese
1 each Chipolte Chile, soaked and finely chopped
1 Tbsp basil, chopped

1. Bring stock to boil and slowly add polenta while whisking.
2. Turn heat down to simmer and cook slowly for 15 minutes.
3. Stir in oil, parmesan, Chipolte, and basil.

Spicy Sprouts with Garlic

2 tsp garlic, chopped
1 tsp safflower oil
2 cup bean sprouts, washed
1 tsp Braggs Liquid Aminos
1/4 tsp red pepper flakes

1. In a non-stick skillet heat oil on low and cook garlic lightly
   for one minute.
2. Remove from heat. Toss in sprouts, Aminos and red pepper
   and mix well. Serve.

Roasted Carrots

1 lb whole carrots
1 Tbsp raw honey
1 tsp tarragon, chopped

1. Wash and split carrots length wise. Cook at 400 for 15 minutes, while rotating pan twice during cooking.
2. Remove carrots from oven and toss with honey and tarragon.

Roasted Tomato Salsa

2 lbs tomatoes, washed and stemmed
1/4 cup basil leaves

1. Roast tomatoes in a pre-heated 400° oven for 1/2 hour.
2. Let tomatoes cool for 15 minutes. Add them to a blender and puree.
3. Add basil and serve hot or cold.

Cornmeal Crusted Catfish w/ Tartar Sauce

2 6-ounce catfish filets
1 Tbsp Dijon Mustard
¼ cup corn grits
1 recipe tartar sauce

1. Spread Mustard on top of catfish filets evenly. Cover filets with corn grits and bake at 350° for 12 minutes.
2. Remove and serve with tartar sauce.

Mustard Basil Salmon

1 tsp garlic, chopped
1 tsp basil, chopped
¼ cup Dijon mustard
2 6-ounce wild salmon filets

1. Mix garlic and basil. Coat top of salmon with mustard and bake at 325° for 15 minutes.

Shrimp w/ Tomatoes and Garlic

12 ounces medium sized peeled shrimp
1 tsp garlic, chopped
1 cup tomatoes, ½ inch diced
¼ cup organic white wine
1 Tbsp basil, chopped
1 Tbsp parsley, chopped
1 Tbsp extra-virgin olive oil

1. Place shrimp, garlic, tomatoes, and wine in a covered casserole dish and bake at 350° for 15 minutes.
2. Remove shrimp from oven and add basil, parsley and oil, serve.

VIII. TOFU, TEMPEH, AND OTHER PROTEINS

Blackened Tofu

1 lb firm tofu
1 Tbsp Cajun seasoning (non-irradiated)
1 recipe Roasted tomato Salsa.

1. Slice tofu into four equal pieces. Let tofu drain wrapped in towel for 20 minutes.
2. Spread Cajun seasoning on a plate and cover one or both sides of tofu (depends on how spicy you like it).
3. Heat a medium non-stick skillet on medium-high heat. Place tofu in skillet and sear each side until a desired degree of color is reached.
4. Serve with Roasted Tomato Salsa.

Curried Mushroom and Tofu Gratin

1/2 cup TVP (textured vegetable protein)
2 tsp safflower oil
1 tsp garlic, chopped
1/2 cup onions, 1/2 inch diced
3 cups mushrooms, washed, stems removed, and sliced
1 tsp Madras Curry powder
1/2 lb firm tofu, drained and crumbled

1. In a food processor pulse TVP to the consistency of bread crumbs, reserve.
2. Heat oil in a non-stick skillet on low. Cook onions, garlic and mushrooms on low for ten minutes, until mushrooms are cooked and moisture has cooked off.
3. Add curry, tofu and cook on low for ten more minutes.
4. Put mixture in a casserole dish and top with TVP.
5. Bake at 350 for 20 minutes until TVP has browned.

Tempeh Marinara with Rice Penne

8 ounces Tempeh, crumbled
1 cup marinara sauce (see basic recipes)
1/2 lb rice penne
2 Tbsp extra-virgin olive oil

1. Add Tempeh to marinara sauce and bring to a simmer.
2. Cook penne according to labels directions. Toss penne with marinara and olive oil and serve.

Marinara

1 Tbsp safflower oil
1 medium onion medium ½ inch dice
4 cloves garlic chopped
1 sprig thyme
1 bay leaf
¼ cup balsamic vinegar
1 28 oz can of crushed tomatoes

1. Gently cook onion in oil in a thick bottom saucepot.
2. Add vinegar and reduce by half.
3. Add garlic, thyme, bay leaves and tomatoes.
4. Simmer for 15 minutes and serve or cool for later use.

Chef Notes:
This is basic marinara sauce. You may add olives, mushrooms, ground soy meat and/or vegetables.

IX. MISCELLANEOUS

Spinach Lasagna

1 Tbsp safflower oil
½ cup onion, ¼ inch diced
1 tsp garlic, chopped
1 lb firm tofu, drained and crumbled
1 cup cooked and chopped spinach
3 cups marinara
½ box rice lasagna (no boil)
¼ cup vegan parmesan, shredded
¼ cup vegan mozzarella, shredded

1. Heat oil on low heat in a large skillet. Cook onion and garlic for five minutes and add tofu. Cook tofu for ten minutes on low heat. Add spinach and half of the marinara and heat throughout.
2. In a 9 by 9 glass baking dish layer marinara, noodles, tofu and repeat. Top with cheese and cover.
3. Bake at 350° for one hour.

Yukon Mashed Potatoes with Mushroom Sauce

1 lb medium Yukon Potatoes
1 sprig thyme
1 sprig rosemary
1 each bay leaf
1/4 cup plain rice milk
to taste freshly ground white pepper

MUSHROOM SAUCE:
1 Tbsp safflower oil
1 tsp garlic, chopped
1/4 cup onion, 1/4 inch diced
1 1/2 cups assorted mushroom (shiitakes, white, oyster, portobello,
   crimini, chanterelle etc.)
1 tsp tarragon chopped
1 recipe Demi-glace

FOR THE SAUCE:
1. Heat oil in a sauce pan on low. Cook garlic and onion until transparent.
2. Add mushrooms and cook on low for 15 minutes.
3. Add tarragon and Demi-glace. Hold for potatoes.

FOR THE POTATOES:
1. Wash and half the potatoes. Place them in a pot of cold water with thyme, rosemary and bay leaf. Bring potatoes to a simmer and cook for approximately 30 minutes. Insert a knife into potatoes to test doneness.
2. Drain potatoes and pass them through a ricer. Add rice milk and pepper.
3. Serve potatoes with Mushroom Sauce.

X. DESSERTS

Baked Bananas and Berries

2 to 3 bananas
1 cup mixed berries (any combination)
2 Tbsp maple syrup
1/8 tsp ground cinnamon
1/4 cup pecans

1. Peel bananas and place them in a small casserole dish with berries. Top with maple syrup, cinnamon and pecans.
2. Bake covered at 350 for 20 minutes. Serve warm alone or with Rice Dream™.

Chocolate Pudding

2 cups rice milk
2 tsp agar flakes
3/4 cup succanat (evaporated cane juice)
1/3 cup cocoa powder
1 Tbsp coconut oil
2 Tbsp arrowroot dissolved in 2 Tbsp of water

1. Simmer rice milk and agar flakes for about five minutes until dissolved. Add succanat, cocoa powder and coconut oil and simmer for two more minutes.
2. Stir in arrowroot while simmering. Remove and chill for two hours. Puree until smooth and serve with fresh fruit.

Sautéed Strawberries with Rice Dream™

1 pint strawberries, washed and halved
1 each vanilla bean, split and scraped (1 tsp vanilla extract)
⅛ tsp ground cinnamon
1 Tbsp brown rice syrup
Vanilla Rice Dream

1. Heat a non-stick sauté pan on low heat. Add Strawberries and cook for three minutes. Add vanilla, cinnamon and rice syrup and continue to cook on low until strawberries for another three minutes.
2. Serve over Rice Dream.

Vegan Demi Glace

2 cups pomegranate juice
2 sprigs thyme
1 sprig rosemary
2 cups vegetarian beef stock
2 Tbsp arrowroot

1. Put pomegranate juice, thyme, and rosemary in a saucepan and reduce by three-quarters.
2. Add stock and bring to a simmer.
3. Mix arrowroot with 2 Tbsp of water. Add arrowroot to sauce while stirring.
4. Allow to simmer for 2 more minutes and strain.

7

TESTIMONIALS

AFTER years of conducting support groups and studies that had specific considerations, such as arthritis, we have gathered positive statistical analyses of bio-markers pertinent to these conditions. I asked a few of my graduates to make comments about their support group results for this book.

Gayle
I decided to try a disciplined Gary Null protocol because my life was a wheel of pain.

I had migraine headaches, arthritis, bursitis, and tendonitis.

It was a pleasure meeting other people who had long-term conditions. I basked in their friendship and cooperation. We all were on a road together.

Today I am organic and use green and red powders. I read labels and enjoy organic vegan food. It took some time and many homework assignments, (which were tough at times, but I did them).

I no longer suffer from the above-mentioned conditions. I feel younger and much happier.

Dorothy
When I joined the Gary Null support group I had arthritis and was overweight, fatigued, and frequently overslept. I did not know

a thing about healthy living and thinking and never heard the term "toxic people." I was there to learn and improve myself.

Juicing, being organic, vegetarianism, giving up dairy and sodas and sweets seemed alien to me but when I look back I was the alien, not living to my full potential. This experience changed my outlook and taught me a lot.

I do not have arthritis pain. I lost a good deal of weight.

All this made me an energetic, vital person. I do not need to sleep as much because my body is younger and free of allergies and toxins.

Carol

I was arthritic and could not get into or out of a car or stand correctly. My energy sank. I had large moles on my skin.

I joined a support group in 1997. I can honestly say I no longer have symptoms of arthritis. I exercise, do yoga and joined a rowing team. I won several medals with my team.

I lost 65 pounds. The skin moles flattened out. I am energetic and active. I am also quite happy.

Nina

I was diagnosed with lung cancer. I was anemic, had arthritis, almost no energy, and elevated blood pressure. Pain went through me when I walked. I underwent radiation, chemotherapy, body scans.

I was ready for a life change but was not certain where to go or whom to see. After hearing Gary Null on television and radio I was curious and joined a health support group.

I ate flesh foods and dairy. Today I am vegan. I drink green juices and follow the protocol totally. I am cancer free without medication. My arthritis has diminished and I can use and enjoy my body by walking, doing yoga, and working in the wardrobe department of a theatrical company. I look forward to a good season with the crew. I am delighted with the results of each new blood test. The class homework motivated me to go forward, made me understand myself and my former pitfalls. I developed personal insight.

Pat

"I am a walking miracle." I weighed 225 pounds. I was hospitalized three times for congestive heart disease. I also suffered from arthritis, diabetes, sciatica, and glaucoma.

I lived in a wheelchair 24 hours a day on oxygen using steroids for emphysema. It was in this condition that I was wheeled into the Los Angeles Gary Null health support group to turn this unhappy life around.

Today I am not in pain from arthritis or discomfort with emphysema. I take long walks daily. I am an organic vegan carefully keeping to the protocol that revitalized my life.

I lost weight and most of all I lost contact with the toxic situations and people that formerly kept me in the sick mode.

Shelly

I felt the effects of what I thought was aging and was quite despondent. I was usually fatigued, had arthritis, high blood pressure and cholesterol. I was diagnosed with cataracts, osteoporosis, and obesity. My hair and nails were weak. This made me sensitive to the opinions of others.

I followed my new food and lifestyle protocol carefully and can proudly say "I did it." things are much happier today.

I lost twenty pounds. My hair and nails are growing stronger. I look younger. I do not have aches and pains nor am I tired most of the time.

My indifference to criticism is just one major step to my new life. My husband accepted a job on the west coast, a change that would have upset me years ago. Today I look forward to his visits and my trips to see him. It is exciting.

Thomas, 70 years old

I was very interested in Gary Null's radio guests. Some of the people began their juicing and organic protocol because they had illnesses. They spoke about belonging to a group that gave them the strength to change. I needed that.

I am a Parkinson's patient. I had hypertension, b simplex outbreaks, arthritis and skin problems. I became aware of the importance of nutrition and studied various theories but my physical problems continued. Parkinson symptoms caused shame in public. I could not write and I typed with two fingers. My hands trembled when I put food in my mouth.

I was prescribed medications but past experiences were unpleasant so I refused them. I began Gary's detoxification protocol and learned the specifics of diet and organics; the biochemical necessity of green juices and grasses; the importance of attitude and beliefs.

Things began to look up. I now honor myself, unclutter my life of people and objects and share my knowledge with others. I am alert without past negative influences. Green and red drinks keep me going. These are my happiest and proudest times. I intend to live another seventy years.

Warnetta, 82 years old

I listened to Gary's show many years before I actualized the information. My cholesterol and blood pressure were elevated but my primary concern was obesity—my weight was 209. I wore a size 22 and was diagnosed with an underactive thyroid, low energy, osteoporosis, osteoarthritis, cataracts, and carpal tunnel syndrome. Gary explained detoxification must precede dieting to be effective. That made a lot of sense to me so I went with the protocol.

Today I weigh 150 pounds and maintain it. Recent physical examinations ruled out an abnormal thyroid, carpal tunnel syndrome and cataracts. I take lutein and blueberry capsules and threaded a fine needle today without difficulty. My cholesterol and blood pressure are slightly elevated but not abnormal. I have no symptoms of osteoarthritis or osteoporosis.

I exercise three times a week with a senior class in a Buddhist temple. I buy organic food, stopped eating meat and eat fish. Ingredient labels shocked me. I am more aware of the unnecessary amount of salt in products. I explain these concepts to people interested in regaining their health. I am determined to enjoy life in good health and with positive energy.

Monique

The support group changed my life and health. I am very pleased with my results. I had a hysterectomy to remove uterine cancer. The cancer returned. I underwent chemotherapy and radiation. I also had arthritis, psoriasis, low energy, obesity and was unhappy at work.

I sought a new experience, a new route to health. After listening to Gary Null on the air and listening to people who changed their lives and health following his protocol I joined a health support group.

Today I am vegan and organic. I follow the protocol. I use green juices and organic food. I take supplements. My cancer seems to be in full remission. I am 26 pounds thinner. The psoriasis is gone my hair and skin are healthy and the arthritis is gone. My immune system is strong.

It was through class assignments and other workbook activities that I understood how hard I was on myself and soon experienced the positive relief of forgiveness. Best of all, I left my toxic job. I meditate twice daily, exercise, practice yoga and lift weights.

Tom

I really felt I was getting old. Excess weight, skin problems, arthritis, fatigue, eyesight failing, hearing not as acute as it was, all these were depressing. My cholesterol and blood pressure were high.

I had nothing to lose. Gary was a health expert and there was no reason I could not achieve what others did on his program. I went into a support group and had really good results.

As I followed the vegan, organic program I lost 30 pounds which increased my energy. My skin began to look better and better. Arthritis in my joints lessened and is now gone. My eyesight and hearing improved and the cholesterol and blood pressure values are normal

There is every reason to spread the word. If it happened to me anyone can regain their health.

REFERENCES

CHAPTER THREE

1. *"Super-aspirin is turning out to be a super-failure, perhaps even a deadly one."* Seattle Times, January 29, 2000.
2. Susan Okie. "Sharp Rise Reported in Multiple Prescriptions." *Washington Post*, July 18, 2001, p. A02.
3. *New York Times*, May 8, 2001.
4. National Institute for Health Care Management Research and Educational Foundation, May 11, 2001.
5. Anthony A, Dhillon AP, Fidler H, McFadden J, Billington O, Nygard G, Pounder RE, Wakefield AJ. Mycobacterial granulomatous inflammation in the ulcerated caecum of indomethacin-treated rats. Int J Exp Pathol 1995 Apr;76(2):149–55.
6. Keane J, Gershon S, Wise RP, Mirabile-Levens E, Kasznica J, Schwieterman WD, Siegel JN, Braun MM. Tuberculosis associated with infliximab, a tumor necrosis factor alpha-neutralizing agent. *New England Journal of Medicine* October 11, 2001;345(15):1098–1104.
7. *Melody Petersen. New York Times, April 11, 2002.*
8. Bachmeyer C, Vermeulen C, Habki R, Blay F, Leynadier F. Acetaminophen (paracetamol)-induced anaphylactic shock. South Med J. 2002 Jul.95 (7):759–60.
9. Kozer E, Barr J, Bulkowstein M, Avgil M, Greenberg R, Matias A, Petrov I, Berkovitch M. A prospective study of multiple supratherapeutic acetaminophen doses in febrile children. Vet Hum Toxicol. 2002 Apr;44 (2):106–9.
10. Physician's Desk Reference.

References

11. Santucci L, Fiorucci S, Patoia L, Di Matteo FM, Brunori PM, Morelli A. Severe gastric mucosal damage induced by NSAIDs in healthy subjects is associated with Helicobacter pylori infection and high levels of serum pepsinogens. Dig Dis Sci 1995 Sep;40(9):2074–80.

12. New England Journal of Medicine. June 2000.

13. Antonicelli L, Tagliabracci A. Asthma death induced by ibuprofen. Monaldi Arch Chest Dis. 1995 Aug;50(4):276–8.

14. Butterfield JH, Schwenk NM, Colville DS, Kuipers BJ. Severe generalized reactions to ibuprofen: report of a case. J Rheumatol. 1986 Jun;13 (3):649–50.

15. Askholt J, Nielsen-Kudsk F. Ibuprofen, pharmacokinetics and pharmacodynamics in the isolated rabbit heart. Acta Pharmacol Toxicol (Copenh). 1985 Feb;56(2):99–107.

16. MacAllister CG, Morgan SJ, Borne AT, Pollet RA. Comparison of adverse effects of phenylbutazone, flunixin meglumine, and ketoprofen in horses. J Am Vet Med Assoc. 1993 Jan 1;202(1):71–7.

17. Durieu C, Marguery MC, Giordano-Labadie F, Journe F, Loche F, Bazex J. Photoaggravated contact allergy and contact photoallergy caused by ketoprofen: 19 cases. Ann Dermatol Venereol. 2001 Oct;128(10 Pt 1):1020–4.

18. Le Coz CJ, Bottlaender A, Scrivener JN, Santinelli F, Cribier BJ, Heid E, Grosshans EM. Photocontact dermatitis from ketoprofen and tiaprofenic acid: cross-reactivity study in 12 consecutive patients. Contact Dermatitis. 1998 May;38(5):245–52.

19. Bastien M, Milpied-Homsi B, Baudot S, Dutartre H, Litoux P. Ketoprofen-induced contact photosensitivity disorders: 5 cases. Ann Dermatol Venereol. 1997;124(8):523–6.

20. Sugiura M, Hayakawa R, Xie Z, Sugiura K, Hiramoto K, Shamoto M. Experimental study on phototoxicity and the photosensitization potential of ketoprofen, suprofen, tiaprofenic acid and benzophenone and the photocross-reactivity in guinea pigs. Photodermatol Photoimmunol Photomed. 2002 Apr;18(2):82–9.

21. Laroche F, Kahan A, Kahan A, Letrait M, Cohen C, Jamin P, Strauch G. Ketoprofen and prednisolone do not modulate neutrophil CR1, CR3 and Fc gamma RIII expression in healthy volunteers. Br J Clin Pharmacol. 1994 Nov;38(5):441–5.

22. Gonzalo Garijo MA, Bobadilla Gonzalez P. Cutaneous reaction to naproxen. Allergol Immunopathol (Madr). 1996 Mar-Apr;24(2):89–92.

References

23. Lipscomb GR, Wallis N, Armstrong G, Goodman MJ, Rees WD. Influence of Helicobacter pylori on gastric mucosal adaptation to naproxen in man. Dig Dis Sci. 1996 Aug;41(8):1583–8.

24. Shelley ED, Shelley WB, Burmeister V. Naproxen-induced pseudoporphyria presenting a diagnostic dilemma. Cutis. 1987 Oct;40(4):314–6.

25. Prieto L, Pastor A, Palop A, Castro J, Paricio A, Piquer A. Rhinitis with intolerance to non-steroidal anti-inflammatory agents. Report of 3 cases. Allergol Immunopathol (Madr). 1986 Mar-Apr;14(2):147–53.

26. Bougie D, Aster R. Immune thrombocytopenia resulting from sensitivity to metabolites of naproxen and acetaminophen. Blood. 2001 Jun 15;97 (12):3846–50.

27. Ding C. Do NSAIDs affect the progression of osteoarthritis? Inflammation. 2002 Jun;26(3):139–42.

28. Moreno-Sanchez R, Bravo C, Vasquez C, Ayala G, Silveira LH, Martinez-Lavin M. Inhibition and uncoupling of oxidative phosphorylation by non-steroidal anti-inflammatory drugs: study in mitochondria, submitochondrial particles, cells, and whole heart. Biochem Pharmacol. 1999 Apr 1;57(7): 743–52.

29. Johnson AG. NSAIDs and increased blood pressure. What is the clinical significance? Drug Saf. 1997 Nov;17(5):277–89.

30. Bulstra SK, Kuijer R, Buurman WA, Terwindt-Rouwenhorst E, Guelen PJ, van der Linden AJ. The effect of piroxicam on the metabolism of isolated human chondrocytes. Clin Orthop 1992 Apr;(277):289–96.

31. Serrano G, Bonillo J, Aliaga A, Gargallo E, Pelufo C. Piroxicam-induced photosensitivity. In vivo and in vitro studies of its photosensitizing potential. J Am Acad Dermatol 1984 Jul;11(1):113–20.

32. Trujillo MJ, de Barrio M, Rodriguez A, Moreno-Zazo M, Sanchez I, Pelta R, Tornero P, Herrero T. Piroxicam-induced photodermatitis. Cross-reactivity among oxicams. A case report. Allergol Immunopathol (Madr) 2001 Jul-Aug;29(4):133–6.

33. Goncalo M, Figueiredo A, Tavares P, Ribeiro CA, Teixeira F, Baptista AP. Photosensitivity to piroxicam: absence of cross-reaction with tenoxicam. Contact Dermatitis 1992 Nov;27(5):287–90.

34. Plunkett RW, Chiarello SE, Beutner EH. Linear IgA bullous dermatosis in one of two piroxicam-induced eruptions: a distinct direct immunofluorescence trend revealed by the literature. J Am Acad Dermatol 2001 Nov;45 (5):691–6.

References

35. Poniachik J, Guerrero J, Calderon P, Smok G, Morales A, Munoz G, Venegas M. Cholestatic hepatitis associated with piroxicam use. Case report. Rev Med Chil 1998 May;126(5):548–52.

36. Ordoqui E, De Barrio M, Rodriguez VM, Herrero T, Gil PJ, Baeza ML. Cross-sensitivity among oxicams in piroxicam-caused fixed drug eruption: two case reports. Allergy 1995 Sep;50(9):741–4.

37. Rochon PA et al. A Study of Manufacture-Supported Trials of Nonsteroidal Anti-Inflammatory Drugs in the Treatment of Arthritis. Archives of Internal Medicine 1994; 154:157–63.

38. Fernandez-Rivas M, de la Hoz B, Cuevas M, Davila I, Quirce S, Losada E. Hypersensitivity reactions to anthranilic acid derivatives. Ann Allergy 1993 Dec;71(6):515–8.

39. McGwin G Jr, Sims RV, Pulley L, Roseman JM. Relations among chronic medical conditions, medications, and automobile crashes in the elderly: a population-based case-control study. Am J Epidemiol 2000 Sep 1;152 (5):424–31.

40. Mukherjee D, Nissen SE, Topol EJ. Risk of cardiovascular events associated with selective COX-2 inhibitors. JAMA. 2001 Aug 22–29;286 (8):954–9.

41. British Medical Journal June 1, 2002;324:1287–1290.

42. Washington Post, August 5, 2001, p.A11.

43. Advisory Panel to the U.S. Food and Drug Administration, Gaithersburg, MD, February 8, 2001.

44. Silverstein FE, Faich G, Goldstein JL, Simon LS, Pincus T, Whelton A, Makuch R, Eisen G, Agrawal NM, Stenson WF, Burr AM, Zhao WW, Kent JD, Lefkowith JB, Verburg KM, Geis GS. Gastrointestinal toxicity with celecoxib vs nonsteroidal anti-inflammatory drugs for osteoarthritis and rheumatoid arthritis: the CLASS study: A randomized controlled trial. Celecoxib Long-term Arthritis Safety Study. JAMA 2000 Sep 13;284 (10):1247–55.

45. www.kineretrx.com

46. Ryan ME, Greenwald RA, Golub LM. Potential of tetracyclines to modify cartilage breakdown in osteoarthritis. Curr Opin Rheumatol 1996 May;8(3):238–47.

47. Sieper J, Braun J, Editorial: Treatment of Reactive Arthritis with Antibiotics. British Journal of Rheumatology 1998;37(7):717–720.

References

48. Smith GN Jr, Yu LP Jr, Brandt KD, Capello WN. Oral administration of doxycycline reduces collagenase and gelatinase activities in extracts of human osteoarthritic cartilage. Journal of Rheumatology 1998;25(3): 532–535.

49. Tilley BC, Alarcon GS, Heyse SP, Trentham DE, Neuner R, Kaplan DA, Clegg DO, Leisen JC, Buckley L, Cooper SM, Duncan H, Pillemer SR, Tuttleman M, Fowler SE. Minocycline in rheumatoid arthritis: A 48–week, double-blind, placebo-controlled trial, MIRA Trial Group. Annals of Internal Medicine 1995; 122(2):81–89.

50. Trentham DE, Dynesius-Trentham RA. Antibiotic therapy for rheumatoid arthritis. Scientific and anecdotal appraisals. Rheum Dis Clin North Am 1995 Aug;21(3):817–34.

51. "FDA Approves Amgen's RA Drug," Reuters, November 14, 2001.

52. http://arthritis.about.com/library/weekly/aa111801a.htm

53. http://www.discovercentrus.com

54. Results of the VIGOR study. Rofecoxib halves the complication rate. MMW Fortschr Med 2001 Jun 7;143(23):35.

55. Mukherjee D, Nissen SE, Topol EJ. Risk of cardiovascular events associated with selective COX-2 inhibitors. JAMA 2001 Aug 22–29;286(8): 954–9.

56. Bonnel RA, Villalba ML, Karwoski CB, Beitz J. Aseptic meningitis associated with rofecoxib. Arch Intern Med 2002 Mar 25; 162(6):713–5.

57. Science 2002 April 19; 296:539–541.

58. van Outryve S, Schrijvers D, van den Brande J, Wilmes P, Bogers J, van Marck E, Vermorken JB. Methotrexate-associated liver toxicity in a patient with breast cancer: case report and literature review. Neth J Med. 2002 Jun; 60(5):216–22.

59. Padeh S, Sharon N, Schiby G, Rechavi G, Passwell JH. Hodgkin's lymphoma in systemic onset juvenile rheumatoid arthritis after treatment with low dose methotrexate. J Rheumatol. 1997 Oct; 24(10):2035–7.

60. Falcini F, Taccetti G, Ermini M, Trapani S, Calzolari A, Franchi A, Cerinic MM. Methotrexate-associated appearance and rapid progression of rheumatoid nodules in systemic-onset juvenile rheumatoid arthritis. Arthritis Rheum. 1997 Jan; 40(1):175–8.

61. Roux N, Flipo RM, Cortet B, Lafitte JJ, Tonnel AB, Duquesnoy B, Delcambre B. Pneumocystis carinii pneumonia in rheumatoid arthritis patients

treated with methotrexate. A report of two cases. Rev Rhum Engl Ed. 1996 Jun; 63(6):453–6.

62. Israel CW, Wegener M, Adamek RJ, Bitsch T, Weber K, Ricken D. Severe pneumonitis as a complication of low-dose methotrexate therapy in psoriasis-associated polyarthritis. Dtsch Med Wochenschr. 1995 Apr 28; 120(17):603–8.

63. Arthritis & Rheumatism July 2001; 44:1515–1524.

64. Mirmohammadsadegh A, Homey B, Abts HF, Kohrer K, Ruzicka T, Michel G. Differential modulation of pro- and anti-inflammatory cytokine receptors by N-(4–trifluoromethylphenyl)-2–cyano-3-hydroxy-crotonic acid amide (A771726), the physiologically active metabolite of the novel immuno-modulator leflunomide. Biochem Pharmacol. 1998 May 1; 55(9):1523–9.

65. Shawver LK, Schwartz DP, Mann E, Chen H, Tsai J, Chu L, Taylorson L, Long Hi M, Meredith S, Germain L, Jacobs JS, Tang C, Ullrich A, Berens ME, Hersh E, McMahon G, Hirth KP, Powell TJ. Inhibition of platelet-derived growth factor-mediated signal transduction and tumor growth by N[4–(trifluoromethyl)-phenyl]5–methylisoxazole-4–carboxamide. Clin Cancer Res. 1997 Jul; 3(7):1167–77.

66. Public Citizen, March 28, 2002.

67. Lau G, Kwan C, Chong SM. The 3–week sulphasalazine syndrome strikes again. Forensic Sci Int. 2001 Nov 1; 122(2–3):79–84.

68. Schoonjans R, Mast A, Van den Abeele G, Dewilde D, Achten E, Van Maele V, Pauwels W. Sulfasalazine-associated encephalopathy in a patient with Crohn's disease. Am J Gastroenterol. 1993 Oct; 88(10):1759–63.

69. Knowles SR, Gupta AK, Shear NH, Sauder D. Azathioprine hypersensitivity-like reactions—a case report and a review of the literature. Clin Exp Dermatol. 1995 Jul; 20(4):353–6.

70. Lau JY, Bird GL, Alexander GJ, Williams R. Effects of immunosuppressive therapy on hepatic expression of hepatitis B viral genome and gene products. Clin Invest Med. 1993 Jun; 16(3):226–36.

71. Giacchino R, Facco F, Loy A, Timitilli A, Cirillo C, Navone C, Ciravegna B, Pisani N. Reactivation of virus replication during immunosuppressive therapy in children with chronic hepatitis B. Boll Ist Sieroter Milan. 1989; 68(1):24–7.

72. Ebo DG, Piel GC, Conraads V, Stevens WJ. IgE-mediated anaphylaxis after first intravenous infusion of cyclosporine. Ann Allergy Asthma Immunol 2001 Sep; 87(3):243–5.

References

73. Meier H, Elsner P, Wuthrich B. Occupationally-induced contact dermatitis and bronchial asthma in a unusual delayed reaction to hydroxychloroquine. Hautarzt 1999 Sep; 50(9):665–9.

74. Wijnands MJ, Van 't Hof MA, Van Leeuwen MA, Van Rijswijk MH, Van de Putte LB, Van Riel PL. A prospective analysis of risk factors for the discontinuation of second-line antirheumatic drugs. Pharm World Sci 1993 Oct 15; 15(5):203–7.

75. Garrood T, Scott DL. Combination therapy with disease modifying antirheumatic drugs in rheumatoid arthritis. BioDrugs. 2001; 15(8):543–61.

76. Verhoeven AC, Boers M, Tugwell P. Combination therapy in rheumatoid arthritis: updated systematic review. Br J Rheumatol. 1998 Jun; 37(6): 612–9.

77. Massone C, Parodi A, Virno G, Rebora A. Multiple eruptive dermatofibromas in patients with systemic lupus erythematosus treated with prednisone. Int J Dermatol 2002 May; 41(5):279–81.

78. Alegre-Sancho JJ, Juanola X, Narvaez FJ, Roig-Escofet D. Septic arthritis due to Prevotella bivia in a patient with rheumatoid arthritis. Joint Bone Spine 2000; 67(3):228–9.

79. Fiter J, Nolla JM, Navarro MA, Gomez-Vaquero C, Rosel P, Mateo L, Roig-Escofet D. Weak androgen levels, glucocorticoid therapy, and bone mineral density in postmenopausal women with rheumatoid arthritis. Joint Bone Spine 2000; 67(3):228–9.

80. Ringe JD. Generalized osteoporosis in chronic polyarthritis-pathomechanisms and treatment approaches. J Clin Oncol 1996 Jun; 14(6):1943–9.

81. Laan RF, van Riel PL, van Erning LJ, Lemmens JA, Ruijs SH, van de Putte LB. Vertebral osteoporosis in rheumatoid arthritis patients: effect of low dose prednisone therapy. Rev Rhum Mal Osteoartic 1992 May; 59(5): 303–9.

82. Schacht E. Osteoporosis in rheumatoid arthritis—significance of alfacalcidol in prevention and therapy. Proc Natl Acad Sci U S A 2000 May 9; 97(10):5645–50.

83. Mauras N. Growth hormone therapy in the glucocorticosteroid-dependent child: metabolic and linear growth effects. Inflamm Bowel Dis 2002 May; 8(3):186–91.

84. Kotaniemi A, Savolainen A, Kroger H, Kautiainen H, Isomaki H. Weight-bearing physical activity, calcium intake, systemic glucocorticoids, chronic inflammation, and body constitution as determinants of lumbar and

femoral bone mineral in juvenile chronic arthritis. Z Rheumatol 2000; 59 Suppl 1:10–20.

85. Armstrong RW, Bolding F. Septic arthritis after arthroscopy: the contributing roles of intraarticular steroids and environmental factors. Am J Infect Control. 1994 Feb; 22(1):16–8.

86. Nakamura H, Yoshino S, Ishiuchi N, Fujimori J, Kanai T, Nishimura Y. Outcome of radical multiple synovectomy as a novel surgical treatment for refractory rheumatoid arthritis: implication of HLA-DRB1*0405 in postoperative results. Clin Exp Rheumatol. 1997 Jan-Feb; 15(1):53–7.

87. Sypniewska G, Lis K, Bilinski PJ. Bone turnover markers and cytokines in joint fluid: analyses in 10 patients with loose hip prosthesis and 39 with coxarthrosis. Acta Orthop Scand. 2002 Oct; 73(5):518–22.

88. Takatori Y, Ninomiya S, Umeyama T, Yamamoto M, Moro T, Nakamura K. Bipolar revision arthroplasty for failed threaded acetabular components: radiographic evaluation of cup migration. J Orthop Sci. 2002; 7(4): 467–71.

89. Stephens MA, Druley JA, Zautra AJ. Older adults' recovery from surgery for osteoarthritis of the knee: psychosocial resources and constraints as predictors of outcomes. Health Psychol. 2002 Jul; 21(4):377–83.

90. Ivancevic V, Perka C, Hasart O, Sandrock D, Munz DL, Ivaneeviae V. Imaging of low-grade bone infection with a technetium-99m labelled monoclonal anti-NCA-90 Fab' fragment in patients with previous joint surgery. Eur J Nucl Med Mol Imaging. 2002 Apr; 29(4):547–51.

91. Sarda L, Saleh-Mghir A, Peker C, Meulemans A, Cremieux AC, Le Guludec D. Evaluation of (99m)Tc-ciprofloxacin scintigraphy in a rabbit model of Staphylococcus aureus prosthetic joint infection. J Nucl Med. 2002 Feb; 43(2):239–45.

92. Beaule PE, Campbell P, Mirra J, Hooper JC, Schmalzried TP. Osteolysis in a cementless, second generation metal-on-metal hip replacement. Clin Orthop. 2001 May; (386):159–65.

93. Hirakawa K, Stulberg BN, Wilde AH, Bauer TW, Secic M. Results of 2–stage reimplantation for infected total knee arthroplasty. J Arthroplasty. 1998 Jan; 13(1):22–8.

94. Prats E, Banzo J, Abos MD, Garcia-Lopez F, Escalera T, Garcia-Miralles M, Gaston R, Asenjo MJ. Diagnosis of prosthetic vascular graft infection by technetium-99m-HMPAO-labeled leukocytes. J Nucl Med. 1994 Aug; 35(8):1303–7.

References

95. Windsor RE, Insall JN, Urs WK, Miller DV, Brause BD. Two-stage reimplantation for the salvage of total knee arthroplasty complicated by infection. Further follow-up and refinement of indications. J Bone Joint Surg Am. 1990 Feb; 72(2):272–8.
96. Mariani BD, Tuan RS. Advances in the diagnosis of infection in prosthetic joint implants. Mol Med Today. 1998 May; 4(5):207–13.
97. Lazovic D, Carls J, Floel A, Gratz KF. The value of leukocyte scintigraphy in suspected implant infection in patients with chronic polyarthritis. Chirurg. 1997 Nov; 68(11):1181–6.
98. Mortier J, Engelhardt M. Foreign body reaction in carbon fiber prosthesis implantation in the knee joint—case report and review of the literature. Z Orthop Ihre Grenzgeb. 2000 Sep-Oct; 138(5):390–4.
99. Wong DA, Watson AB. Allergic contact dermatitis due to benzalkonium chloride in plaster of Paris. Australas J Dermatol. 2001 Feb; 42(1):33–5.

CHAPTER FOUR

1. Gabriel SE, Crowson CS, O'Fallon WM. Mortality in rheumatoid arthritis: have we made an impact in 4 decades? J Rheumatol 1999 Dec; 26(12): 2529–33.
2. Morbidity and Mortality Weekly Report 2001 May 4; 50:334–336.
3. Morbidity and Mortality Weekly Report 2002 October 25; 51:948–950.
4. Sutton AJ, Muir KR, Mockett S, Fentem P. A case-control study to investigate the relation between low and moderate levels of physical activity and osteoarthritis of the knee using data collected as part of the Allied Dunbar National Fitness Survey. Ann Rheum Dis 2001 Aug; 60(8):756–64.
5. Symmons DP. Epidemiology of rheumatoid arthritis: determinants of onset, persistence, and outcome. Best Pract Res Clin Rheumatol 2002 Dec. 16(5):707–22.
6. Heliovaara M, Aho K, Knekt P, Impivaara O, Reunanen A, Aromaa A. Coffee consumption, rheumatoid factor, and the risk of rheumatoid arthritis. Ann Rheum Dis 2000 Aug; 59(8):631–5.
7. American College of Rheumatology's annual meeting, San Francisco, November 13, 2001.
8. Uhlig T, Hagen KB, Kvien TK. Current tobacco smoking, formal education, and the risk of rheumatoid arthritis. J Rheumatol 1999 Jan; 26(1):47–54.
9. Laing TJ, Schottenfeld D, Lacey JV Jr, Gillespie BW, Garabrant DH, Cooper BC, Heeringa SG, Alcser KH, Mayes MD. Potential risk factors for

References

undifferentiated connective tissue disease among women: implanted medical devices. Am J Epidemiol 2001 Oct 1; 154(7):610–7.

10. Reckner Olsson A, Skogh T, Wingren G. Comorbidity and lifestyle, reproductive factors, and environmental exposures associated with rheumatoid arthritis. Ann Rheum Dis 2001 Oct; 60(10):934–9.

11. British Medical Journal, February 2, 2002; 234:264–267.

12. Crook, William G., et al. The Yeast Connection: A Medical Breakthrough, 1986.

13. Lucas C, Power L. Dietary fat aggravates active RA. Clin. Res. 1981; 29(4):754A.

14. Lucus C, Power L. JAMA 1982, April 9.

15. Skoldstam L. Fasting and vegan diet in rheumatoid arthritis. Scand J Rheumatol 1986; 15(2):219–21.

16. Panush, R. Food-induced allergic arthritis. Arthritis Rheum. 1986; 29(2): 220–226.

17. Hicklin, J. Clin. Allergy 1980; 10:463.

18. Skoldstam L, Larsson L, Lindstrom FD. Effect of fasting and lactovegetarian diet on rheumatoid arthritis. Scand J Rheumatol 1979; 8(4):249–55

19. Seignalet J. Diet, fasting, and rheumatoid arthritis. Lancet 1992 Jan 4; 339(8784):68–9.

20. Bjarnason I, Williams P, So A, Zanelli GD, Levi AJ, Gumpel JM, Peters TJ, Ansell B. Intestinal permeability and inflammation in rheumatoid arthritis: effects of non-steroidal anti-inflammatory drugs. Lancet 1984 Nov 24; 2(8413):1171–4.

21. Jensen B. Foods That Heal. Avery Publishing. 1988.

22. Borek J. Antioxidant health effects of aged garlic extract. J Nutr 2001 Mar; 131(3s):1010S-5S.

23. Steiner M, Li W.Aged garlic extract, a modulator of cardiovascular risk factors: a dose-finding study on the effects of AGE on platelet functions. J Nutr 2001 Mar; 131(3s):980S-4S.

24. Rahman K. Garlic and aging: new insights into an old remedy. Ageing Res Rev 2003 Jan; 2(1):39–56.

25. Linos A, Kaklamani VG, Kaklamani E, Koumantaki Y, Giziaki E, Papazoglou S, Mantzoros CS.Dietary factors in relation to rheumatoid arthritis: a role for olive oil and cooked vegetables? Am J Clin Nutr 1999 Dec; 70(6):1077–82.

References

26. lminen E, Heikkila S, Poussa T, Lagstrom H, Saario R, Salminen S. Female patients tend to alter their diet following the diagnosis of rheumatoid arthritis and breast cancer. Prev Med 2002 May; 34(5):529–35.

27. Buchbinder R, Gingold M, Hall S, Cohen M. Non-prescription complementary treatments used by rheumatoid arthritis patients attending a community-based rheumatology practice. Intern Med J 2002 May-Jun; 32(5–6):208–14.

28. Kjeldsen-Kragh J, Haugen M, Borchgrevink CF, Laerum E, Eek M, Mowinkel P, Hovi K, Forre O. Controlled trial of fasting and one-year vegetarian diet in rheumatoid arthritis. Lancet 1991 Oct 12; 338(8772): 899–902.

29. Kjeldsen-Kragh J, Haugen M, Borchgrevink CF, Forre O. Vegetarian diet for patients with rheumatoid arthritis-status: two years after introduction of the diet. Clin Rheumatol 1994 Sep; 13(3):475–82.

30. Nenonen M, et al. Effects of uncooked vegan food—living food—on RA, a 3-month controlled and randomized study. AJCN 1992; 56:762.

31. Lall SB, Singh B, Gulati K, Seth SD. Role of nutrition in toxic injury. Indian J Exp Biol 1999 Feb; 37(2):109–16.

32. Fang YZ, Yang S, Wu G. Free radicals, antioxidants, and nutrition. Nutrition 2002 Oct; 18(10):872–9.

33. Knekt P, Kumpulainen J, Jarvinen R, Rissanen H, Heliovaara M, Reunanen A, Hakulinen T, Aromaa A. Flavonoid intake and risk of chronic diseases. Am J Clin Nutr 2002 Sep; 76(3):560–8.

34. Kremer, J. Effect of manipulation of dietary fatty acids on clinical manifestations of RA. Lancet 1985; 1:184–87.

35. Gil A. Polyunsaturated fatty acids and inflammatory diseases. Biomed Pharmacother 2002 Oct; 56(8):388–96.

36. Geusens P, Wouters C, Nijs J, Jiang Y, Dequeker J. Long-term effect of omega-3 fatty acid supplementation in active rheumatoid arthritis. A 12–month, double-blind, controlled study. Arthritis Rheum 1994 Jun; 37(6):824–9. Aug; 13(8):479.

37. Das UN. Beneficial effect of EPA and DHA in the management of SLE and its relationship to the cytokine network. Prostaglandins, Leukotrienes, EFAs 1994; 51:207–213.

38. Nielsen GL, Faarvang KL, Thomsen BS, Teglbjaerg KL, Jensen LT, Hansen TM, Lervang HH, Schmidt EB, Dyerberg J, Ernst E. The effects of dietary

References

supplementation with n-3 polyunsaturated fatty acids in patients with rheumatoid arthritis: a randomized, double blind trial. Eur J Clin Invest 1992 Oct; 22(10):687–91.

39. Faarvang KL, Nielsen GL, Thomsen BS, Teglbjaerg KL, Hansen TM, Lervang HH, Schmidt EB, Dyerberg J, Ernst E. Fish oils and rheumatoid arthritis. A randomized and double-blind study. Ugeskr Laeger 1994 Jun 6; 156(23):3495–8.

40. Rossetti RG, Seiler CM, Laposata M, Zurier RB. Differential regulation of human T lymphocyte protein kinase C activity by unsaturated fatty acids. Clin Immunol Immunopathol 1995 Sep; 76(3 Pt 1):220–4.

41. Darlington LG, Stone TW. Antioxidants and fatty acids in the amelioration of rheumatoid arthritis and related disorders. Br J Nutr 2001 Mar; 85(3): 251–69.

42. Calder PC, Zurier RB. Polyunsaturated fatty acids and rheumatoid arthritis. Curr Opin Clin Nutr Metab Care 2001 Mar; 4(2):115–21.

43. Harrison RA, Harrison BJ. Fish oils are beneficial to patients with established rheumatoid arthritis. J Rheumatol 2001 Nov; 28(11):2563–5.

44. Kremer JM, Lawrence DA, Petrillo GF, Litts LL, Mullaly PM, Rynes RI, Stocker RP, Parhami N, Greenstein NS, Fuchs BR, et al. Effects of high-dose fish oil on rheumatoid arthritis after stopping nonsteroidal anti-inflammatory drugs. Clinical and immune correlates. Arthritis Rheum 1995 Aug; 38(8):1107–14.

45. Gil A. Polyunsaturated fatty acids and inflammatory diseases. Biomed Pharmacother 2002 Oct; 56(8):388–96.

46. Cleland LG, James MJ. Adulthood—prevention: Rheumatoid arthritis. Med J Aust 2002 Jun 3; 176(11 Suppl):S119–20.

47. Gruenwald J, Graubaum HJ, Harde A. Effect of cod liver oil on symptoms of rheumatoid arthritis. Adv Ther 2002 Mar-Apr; 19(2):101–7.

48. Simopoulos AP. Omega-3 Fatty acids in inflammation and autoimmune diseases. J Am Coll Nutr 2002 Dec; 21(6):495–505.

49. Venkatraman J, Meksawan K. Effects of dietary omega3 and omega6 lipids and vitamin E on chemokine levels in autoimmune-prone MRL/MpJ-lpr/lpr mice. J Nutr Biochem 2002.

50. Hansen TM, Lerche A, Kassis V, Lorenzen I, Sondergaard J. Treatment of rheumatoid arthritis with prostaglandin E1 precursors cis-linoleic acid and gamma-linolenic acid. Scand J Rheumatol 1983; 12(2):85–8.

References

51. Horrobin DF. Effects of evening primrose oil in rheumatoid arthritis. Ann Rheum Dis 1989 Nov; 48(11):965–6.

52. Horrobin DF. Essential fatty acid and prostaglandin metabolism in Sjogren's syndrome, systemic sclerosis and rheumatoid arthritis. Scand J Rheumatol Suppl 1986; 61:242–5.

53. Leventhal LJ, Boyce EG, Zurier RB.Treatment of rheumatoid arthritis with gammalinolenic acid. Ann Intern Med 1993 Nov 1; 119(9):867–73.

54. Rothman D, DeLuca P, Zurier RB. Botanical lipids: effects on inflammation, immune responses, and rheumatoid arthritis. Semin Arthritis Rheum 1995 Oct; 25(2):87–96.

55. Zurier RB, Rossetti RG, Jacobson EW, DeMarco DM, Liu NY, Temming JE, White BM, Laposata M. Gamma-Linolenic acid treatment of rheumatoid arthritis. A randomized, placebo-controlled trial. Arthritis Rheum 1996 Nov; 39(11):1808–17.

56. Belch JJ, Hill A. Evening primrose oil and borage oil in rheumatologic conditions. Am J Clin Nutr 2000 Jan; 71(1 Suppl):352S-6S.

57. Kast RE. Borage oil reduction of rheumatoid arthritis activity may be mediated by increased cAMP that suppresses tumor necrosis factor-alpha. Int Immunopharmacol 2001 Nov; 1(12):2197–9.

58. El-Ghobarey, A. Perna canaliculus. Quart. J. Med. 1978; 47:385.

59. Gibson, R. Perna canaliculus in the reaction of arthritis. Practitioner 1980 Sept; 224:955–60. Lancet 1981; 1:439.

60. Felter H W, Lloyd J U. King's American Dispensatory, Vol I and II. Portland, OR. Eclectic Medical Publications, 1983.

61. Mitchell W. Naturopathic Applications of the Botanical Remedies. Seattle, WA. Self-published. 1983.

62. Ellingwood F. Ellingwood's Therapeutics: American Materia Medica Therapeutics and Pharmacognosy. Evanston, IL. 1919.

63. Mitchell W. Naturopathic Applications of the Botanical Remedies. Seattle, WA. Self-published. 1983.

64. Weiss R F. Herbal Medicine. Beaconsfield, England. Beaconsfield Publishers. 1988.

65. Leblan D, Chantre P, Fournie B. Harpagophytum procumbens in the treatment of knee and hip osteoarthritis. Four-month results of a prospective, multicenter, double-blind trial versus diacerhein. Joint Bone Spine 2000; 67(5):462–7.

References

66. British Herbal Pharmacopoeia, p.198.

67. Symphytum officinale (toxic) (leaf): rheumatic pain, arthritis. British Herbal Medical Association. British Herbal Pharmacopoeia, West Yorks, England, 1983.

68. McQuade A L, Hoffman D L. Herbs, Actions and Systems. 1987.

69. Srimal R, Dhawan B. J Pharm Pharmacol 1973; 25:447–52.

70. Srivastava KC and Mustafa T. Med Hypothesis 1992; 39:342–348.

71. Altman RD, Marcussen KC. Effects of a ginger extract on knee pain in patients with osteoarthritis. Arthritis Rheum 2001 Nov; 44(11):2531–8.

72. Schmid B, Ludtke R, Selbmann HK, Kotter I, Tschirdewahn B, Schaffner W, Heide L. Efficacy and tolerability of a standardized willow bark extract in patients with osteoarthritis: randomized placebo-controlled, double blind clinical trial. Phyt other Res 2001 Jun; 15(4):344–50.

73. Schmid B, Ludtke R, Selbmann HK, Kotter I, Tschirdewahn B, Schaffner W, Heide L. Effectiveness and tolerance of standardized willow bark extract in arthrosis patients. Randomized, placebo controlled double-blind study. Z Rheumatol 2000 Oct; 59(5):314–20.

74. Chrubasik S, Eisenberg E, Balan E, Weinberger T, Luzzati R, Conradt C. Treatment of low back pain exacerbations with willow bark extract: a randomized double-blind study. Am J Med 2000 Jul; 109(1):9–14.

75. Bingham, R. Yucca saponin in the management of arthritis. J. Applied Nutr. 1975; 27:45–50.

76. Jung YB, Roh KJ, Jung JA, Jung K, Yoo H, Cho YB, Kwak WJ, Kim DK, Kim KH, Han CK. Effect of SKI 306X, a new herbal anti-arthritic agent, in patients with osteoarthritis of the knee: a double-blind placebo controlled study. AmJ Chin Med 2001; 29(3–4):485–91.

77. Choi JH, Choi JH, Kim DY, Yoon JH, Youn HY, Yi JB, Rhee HI, Ryu KH, Jung K, Han CK, Kwak WJ, Cho YB. Effects of SKI 306X, a new herbal agent, on proteoglycan degradation in cartilage explant culture and collagenase-induced rabbit osteoarthritis model. Osteoarthritis Cartilage 2002 Jun; 10(6):471–8.

78. van Haselen RA, Fisher PA. A randomized controlled trial comparing topical piroxicam gel with a homeopathic gel in osteoarthritis of the knee. Rheumatology (Oxford) 2000 Jul; 39(7):714–9.

79. Lopes Vaz A. Double-blind clinical evaluation of the relative efficacy of ibuprofen and glucosamine sulphate in the management of osteoarthrosis of the knee in out-patients. Curr Med Res Opin 1982; 8(3):145–9.

References

80. Rovati LC, Setnikar I. Glucosamine sulfate compared to ibuprofen in osteoarthritis of the knee. Osteoarthritis Cartilage 1994 Mar; 2(1):61–9. Drug Ther Bull 2002 Nov; 40(11):81–3.

81. Noack W, Fischer M, Forster KK, Rovati LC, Setnikar I. Glucosamine sulfate in osteoarthritis of the knee. Osteoarthritis Cartilage 1994 Mar; 2(1):51–9.

82. Muller-Fassbender H, Bach GL, Haase W, Rovati LC, Setnikar I. Glucosamine sulfate compared to ibuprofen in osteoarthritis of the knee. Osteoarthritis Cartilage 1994 Mar; 2(1):61–9.

83. Reichelt A, Forster KK, Fischer M, Rovati LC, Setnikar I. Efficacy and safety of intramuscular glucosamine sulfate in osteoarthritis of the knee. A randomised, placebo-controlled, double-blind study. Arzneimittelforschung 1994; 44(1):75–80.

84. Qiu GX, Gao SN, Giacovelli G, Rovati L, Setnikar I. Efficacy and safety of glucosamine sulfate versus ibuprofen in patients with knee osteoarthritis. Arzneimittelforschung 1998 May; 48(5):469–74.

85. Pavelka K, Gatterova J, Olejarova M, Machacek S, Giacovelli G, Rovati LC. Glucosamine sulfate use and delay of progression of knee osteoarthritis: a 3–year, randomized, placebo-controlled, double-blind study. Arch Intern Med 2002 Oct 14; 162(18):2113–23.

86. Thie NM, Prasad NG, Major PW. Evaluation of glucosamine sulfate compared to ibuprofen for the treatment of temporomandibular joint osteoarthritis: a randomized double blind controlled 3 month clinical trial. J Rheumatol 2001 Jun; 28(6):1347–55.

87. Reginster JY, Deroisy R, Rovati LC, Lee RL, Lejeune E, Bruyere O, Giacovelli G, Henrotin Y, Dacre JE, Gossett C. Long-term effects of glucosamine sulphate on osteoarthritis progression: a randomised, placebo-controlled clinical trial. Lancet 2001 Jan 27; 357(9252):251–6.

88. Is glucosamine worth taking for osteoarthritis? Drug Ther Bull 2002 Nov; 40(11):81–3.

89. Mazieres B, Loyau G, Menkes CJ, Valat JP, Dreiser RL, Charlot J, Masounabe-Puyanne A. Chondroitin sulfate in the treatment of gonarthrosis and coxarthrosis. 5–months result of a multicenter double-blind controlled prospective study using placebo. Rev Rhum Mal Osteoartic 1992 Jul-Sep; 59(7–8):466–72.

90. Uebelhart D, Thonar EJ, Delmas PD, Chantraine A, Vignon E. Effects of oral chondroitin sulfate on the progression of knee osteoarthritis: a pilot study. Osteoarthritis Cartilage 1998 May; 6 Suppl A:39–46.

References

91. Bucsi L, Poor G. Efficacy and tolerability of oral chondroitin sulfate as a symptomatic slow-acting drug for osteoarthritis (SYSADOA) in the treatment of knee osteoarthritis. Osteoarthritis Cartilage 1998 May; 6 Suppl A:31–6.

92. Bourgeois P, Charles G, Dehais J, Delcambre B, Kuntz JL, Rozenberg S. Efficacy and tolerability of chondroitin sulfate 1200 mg/day vs chondroitin sulfate 3 ¥ 400 mg/day vs placebo. Osteoarthritis Cartilage 1998 May; 6 Suppl A:25–30.

93. Deal CL, Moskowitz RW. Nutraceuticals as therapeutic agents in osteoarthritis. The role of glucosamine, chondroitin sulfate, and collagen hydrolysate. Rheum Dis Clin North Am 1999 May; 25(2):379–95.

94. Nguyen P, Mohamed SE, Gardiner D, Salinas T. A randomized double-blind clinical trial of the effect of chondroitin sulfate and glucosamine hydrochloride on temporomandibular joint disorders: a pilot study. Cranio 2001 Apr; 19(2):130–9.

95. The Journal of the American Medical Association 2000 March 15; 283:1469–1475, 1483–1484.

96. McAlindon T, Felson DT. Nutrition: risk factors for osteoarthritis. Ann Rheum Dis 1997 Jul; 56(7):397–400.

97. Paredes S, Girona J, Hurt-Camejo E, Vallve JC, Olive S, Heras M, Benito P, Masana L. Antioxidant vitamins and lipid peroxidation in patients with rheumatoid arthritis: association with inflammatory markers. J Rheumatol 2002 Nov; 29(11):2271–7.

98. Traver, R.L., et al. Boron and Arthritis: The results of a Double Blind Pilot Study. J of Nut Med 1990; 1:127–32.

99. Kaufman W. J. Am. Geriat. Soc. 1955; 3:927.

100. Nelson MN et al. Proc Soc. Experience. Biol. 1950; 73:31.

101. Barton-Wright EC, Elliott WA. The pantothenic acid metabolism of rheumatoid arthritis. Lancet 1963; 2:862–63.

102. Calcium pantothenate in arthritic conditions. A report from the General Practitioner Research Group. Practitioner 1980; 224:208–11.

103. Bland JH, Cooper SM. A review of the cell biology involved and evidence for reversibility. Management rationally related to known genesis and pathophysiology. Seminars in Arthritis & Rheum. 1984; 14(2):106–33.

104. Schwartz ER. The modulation of osteoarthritic development by vitamins C and E. Int. J. Vit. & Nutr. Research. 1984; Suppl.26:141–6.

105. Prins APA et al. Effect of purified growth factors on rabbit articular chon-

References

drocyte in monolayer culture. Sulfated proteoglycan synthesis. Arthritis Rheum. 1982; 25:1228–38.

106. Krystal G et al. Stimulationof DNA synthesis by ascorbate in culture of articular chondrocytes. Arthritis Rheum. 1982; 25:318–25.

107. Mullen A, Wilson CWM. The metabolism of ascorbic acid in rheumatoid arthritis. Proc. Nutr. Sci. 1976; 35:8A-9A.

108. Sahud MA, Cohen RJ. Effect of aspirin ingestion on ascorbic-acid levels in rheumatoid arthritis. Lancet 1971; 1:937–38.

109. Roberts P, et al. Vitamin C and inflammation. Medicine. Biol. 1984; 62:88.

110. Machtey I, Ouaknine L. Tocopherol in osteoarthritis: A controlled pilot study. J. Am Geriat. Soc. 1978 July; 26(7):328–30.

111. Edmonds SE, Winyard PG, Guo R, Kidd B, Merry P, Langrish-Smith A, Hansen C, Ramm S, Blake DR. Putative analgesic activity of repeated oral doses of vitamin E in the treatment of rheumatoid arthritis. Results of a prospective placebo controlled double blind trial. Ann Rheum Dis 1997 Nov; 56(11):649–55.

112. Simkin, P. Oral zinc sulfate in rheumatoid arthritis. Lancet 1976; 2:539.

113. Clemmensen OJ, et al. Psoriatic arthritis treated with oral zinc sulphate. Brit. J. Dermatol. 1980; 103:411–15.

114. Pandey SP et al. Zinc in rheumatoid arthritis. Indian J. Medicine. Research. 1985; 81:618–20.

115. Pfeiffer C. Zinc and Other Micro-Nutrients. Keats Publishing, 1978.

116. Marz, Russell. Medical Nutrition from Marz, 1997, pp.346–347.

117. Hangarter, W. Copper salicylate in RA and rheumatism-like degenerative disease. Med Welt. 1980; 31:1625.

118. Hangarter W. Inflammation 1977; 2:217.

119. Sorenson JRJ. Copper chelates as possible active forms of anti-arthritic agents. J. Medicine. Chemistry. 1976; 19:135.

120. Williams DA, et al. Synthesis and biological evaluation of tetrakisu (acetylsalicylato)-dicopper (II). J. Pharm. Sci. 1976; 65:126.

121. Sorenson JRJ, Hangarter W. Treatment of rheumatoid and degenerative diseases with copper complexes: A review with emphasis on copper-salicylate. Inflammation 1977; 2:317.

122. Bland J. Copper salicylates and complexes in molecular medicine. Int. Clin. Nutr. Rev. 1984; 4(3):130–4.

References

123. Jacka T, et al. Copper salicylate as an anti-inflammatory and analgesic agent in arthritic rats. Life Sci. 1983 Feb 28; 32(9):1023–30.

124. Walker, WE & Keats DM. An investigation of the therapeutic value of the "copper bracelet:" Dermal assimilation of copper in arthritic/rheumatoid conditions. Agents & Actions 1976; 6:454.

125. Johansson Very, et al. Nutritional status in girls with juvenile chronic arthritis. Human Nutr. Clin. Nutr. 1986; 40C:57–67.

126. Tarp U, et al. Low selenium level in severe rheumatoid arthritis. Scand J. Rheumatol. 1978; 7:237–40.

127. Heinle K, Adam A, Gradl M, Wiseman M, Adam O. Selenium concentration in erythrocytes of patients with rheumatoid arthritis. Clinical and laboratory chemistry infection markers during administration of selenium. Med Klin 1997 Sep 15; 92 Suppl 3:29–31.

128. Sullivan MX, Hess WC. Cystine content of finger nails in arthritis. J. Bone & Joint Surg. 1935; 16:185.

129. Neligan AR, Salt HB. Sulphur in rheumatoid arthritis. Lancet 1934; 2:209.

130. Woldenbert SC. The treatment of arthritis with colloidal sulphur. J. Southern Medicine. Assoc. 1935; 28:875–81.

131. Cohen, Goldman. Bromelain Therapy in RA. Pennsyl. Med. J. 1964 June; 67:27–30.

132. L Long, K Soeken, E Ernst. Herbal medicines for the treatment of osteoarthritis: a systematic review. Rheumatology 2001; 7:779–793.

133. Blotman F, Maheu E, Wulwik A, Caspard H, Lopez A. Efficacy and safety of avocado/soybean unsaponifiables in the treatment of symptomatic osteoarthritis of the knee and hip. A prospective, multicenter, three-month, randomized, double-blind, placebo-controlled trial. Rev Rhum Engl Ed 1997 Dec; 64(12):825–34.

134. Maheu E, Mazieres B, Valat JP, Loyau G, Le Loet X, Bourgeois P, Grouin JM, Rozenberg S. Symptomatic efficacy of avocado/soybean unsaponifiables in the treatment of osteoarthritis of the knee and hip. Arthritis & Rheumatism. 1998 Jan; 41(1):81–91.

135. Appelboom T, Schuermans J, Verbruggen G, Henrotin Y, Reginster JY. Symptoms modifying effect of avocado/soybean unsaponifiables (ASU) in knee osteoarthritis. A double blind, prospective, placebo-controlled study. Scand J Rheumatol 2001; 30(4):242–7.

References

136. Elkayam O, Ophir J, Brener S, Paran D, Wigler I, Efron D, Even-Paz Z, Politi Y, Yaron M. Immediate and delayed effects of treatment at the Dead Sea in patients with psoriatic arthritis. Rheumatol Int 2000; 19(3):77–82.
137. Michalsen A, Deuse U, Esch T, Dobos G, Moebus S. Effect of leeches therapy (Hirudo medicinalis) in painful osteoarthritis.